Essentials of
Health Services

3rd Edition

Essentials of
Health Services

3rd Edition

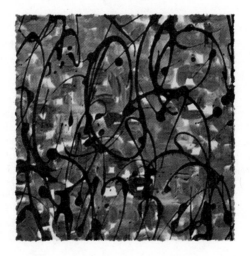

Stephen J. Williams, Sc.D.

Professor of Public Health
Head, Division of Health Services Administration
Graduate School of Public Health
San Diego State University
San Diego, California

THOMSON

DELMAR LEARNING

Australia Canada Mexico Singapore Spain United Kingdom United States

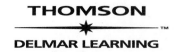

Essentials of Health Services, 3rd Edition
by Stephen J. Williams, Sc.D.

Vice President, Health Care Business Unit:
William Brottmiller

Editorial Director:
Cathy L. Esperti

Acquisitions Editor:
Maureen Rosener

Editorial Assistant:
Elizabeth Howe

Marketing Director:
Jennifer McAvey

Marketing Coordinator:
Michele Gleason

Production Editor:
Bridget Lulay

Library of Congress Cataloging-in-Publication Data
Williams, Stephen J. (Stephen Joseph), 1948-
  Essentials of health services / Stephen J. Williams.-- 3rd ed.
    p. ; cm. -- (Thomson Delmar Learning series in health services administration)
  Includes bibliographical references and index.
  ISBN 1-4018-9931-5
  1. Medical care--United States. 2. Public health--United States. 3. Medical policy--United States.
  [DNLM: 1. Health Services Administration--United States. 2. Delivery of Health Care--United States. 3. Health Planning--United States. 4. Health Policy--United States. W 84 AA1 W64e 2005] I. Title. II. Series.
  RA445.W53 2005
  362.1'0973--dc22
                                    2005000015

Notice to the Reader

This book is dedicated to the memory
of my father,
David Williams.

INTRODUCTION TO THE SERIES

This Series in Health Services is now in its third decade of providing top quality teaching materials to the health administration/public health field. Each year has witnessed further strengthening of the market position of each of the principal books in the series, also reflecting the continued excellence of the products. Each author, book editor, and contributor to the series has helped build what is widely recognized as the top textbook and issues collection of books available in this field today.

But we have achieved only a beginning. Everyone involved in the series is committed to further expansion of the scope, technical excellence, and usability of the series. Our goal is to do more for you, the reader. We will add new books in important areas, seek out more excellent authors, and increase the physical attributes of the books to make them easier for you to use.

We thank everyone, the authors and users in particular, who have made this series so successful and so widely used. And we promise that this third decade will be dedicated to further expansion of the series and to enhancement of the books it contains to provide still greater value to you, our constituency.

Stephen J. Williams
Series Editor

THOMSON DELMAR LEARNING SERIES IN HEALTH SERVICES ADMINISTRATION

Stephen J. Williams, Sc.D., Series Editor

Ambulatory Care Management, 3rd edition
Austin Ross, Stephen J. Williams, and Ernest J. Pavlock, Editors

The Continuum of Long-Term Care, 3rd edition
Connie J. Evashwick, Editor

Health Care Economics, 6th edition
Paul J. Feldstein

Health Politics and Policy, 3rd edition
Theodor J. Litman and Leonard S. Robins, Editors

Introduction to Health Services, 6th edition
Stephen J. Williams and Paul R. Torrens, Editors

Motivating Health Behavior
John P. Elder, E. Scott Geller, Melbourne F. Hovell, and Joni A. Mayer, Editors

Really Governing: How Health System and Hospital Boards Can Make More of a Difference
Dennis D. Pointer and Charles M. Ewell

Strategic Management of Human Resources in Health Services Organizations, 2nd edition
Myron D. Fottler, S. Robert Hernandez, and Charles L. Joiner, Editors

Financial Management in Health Care Organizations, 2nd edition
Robert A. McLean

Principles of Public Health Practice, 2nd edition
F. Douglas Scutchfield and C. William Keck, Editors

The Hospital Medical Staff
Charles H. White

Essentials of Health Services, 3rd edition
Stephen J. Williams

Essentials of Health Care Management
Stephen M. Shortell and Arnold D. Kaluzny, Editors

Essentials of Human Resources Management in Health Services Organizations
Myron D. Fottler, S. Robert Hernandez, and Charles L. Joiner, Editors

Health Services Research Methods
Leiyu Shi

Health Care Management: Organization Design and Behavior, 4th edition
Stephen M. Shortell and Arnold D. Kaluzny, Editors

Contents

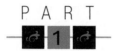

An Overview of Health Care in the United States / 1

P A R T
2
Organizational and Individual Providers / 39

P A R T

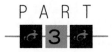

Paying for, Managing, Controlling, and Evaluating the System / 135

PREFACE

This, the third edition of *Essentials of Health Services,* analyzes, describes, and evaluates the nation's health care system. Health care is one of the most important components of our national economic activity, and one of the largest in terms of dollars and other resources. But, ultimately, the nation's health care system is of greatest importance in its contribution to our individual and collective well-being. Our expenditures and investments in health care resources and services serve the ultimate objective of improving how long and how well we live.

The nation's health care system and its interactions and ramifications, as well as the underlying technology that is implemented through the system, has continued to increase dramatically in complexity, cost, and potential contribution to the protection of our life, liberty, and the pursuit of happiness. The economic and political environment within which health care operates has likewise increased in complexity and expectations. Now, more than ever, it is critical for all participants in the health care system, whether we be employed by it, or benefit from its knowledge and service capabilities, to better understand, organize, utilize, evaluate, and enhance the services provided by the system. That, in essence, is the message of this book. How that message is delivered is the subject of the next few paragraphs.

PURPOSE OF THE BOOK

The principal objective of this book is to explain, in relatively straightforward terms, how the nation's health care system is structured and, perhaps more importantly, how it functions. The scope of the system with its many complex and interrelated components is described and analyzed, defined, and illustrated.

This book draws upon, but simplifies, the presentations available in Thomson Delmar Learning's widely acclaimed textbook, *Introduction to Health Services,* 6th edition, edited by Stephen J. Williams and Paul R. Torrens. This text is designed for the more advanced audiences of graduate students in public health, health services administration, and related health professions, and sophisticated practitioners in various fields.

Essentials of Health Services, 3rd edition, seeks to provide a somewhat broader perspective in a format understandable to undergraduate students, to clinicians, and to other individuals with an interest in the increasing role of health care in our nation's society and economy. In this book, particular emphasis is placed on describing and explaining the components of the health care system and on presenting information in an easily readable format.

ORGANIZATION OF MATERIAL

Part 1 of this book provides an overview of the health care system, examines the underlying reasons for health services utilization, and concludes with an examination of the measures used to assess access to health services. Chapter 1, by using historical and financial information, presents an overall perspective on the health care system. Chapter 2 extensively presents the case for how changes in the demographic, sociologic, and economic characteristics of our society lead to the need for health services utilization. Chapter 3 describes measures of access to health care and how we assess the success of individuals in obtaining services.

Part 2 of the book describes and analyzes the settings in which health care services are offered to consumers, and the people and organizations, including the pharmaceutical industry, that participate. The chapters focus on the major categories of providers. Chapter 4 describes in detail the provision of ambulatory care services, which now represents the backbone of the nation's health care system. Chapter 5 provides a perspective on public health services, which still represent our first line of defense against disease and illness. Chapter 6 describes the dramatic changes occurring in the nation's hospitals and health systems, particularly with regard to consolidation and multihospital systems. Chapters 7 and 8 focus on mental health services and long-term care services respectively, both of which are major areas of challenge for the future. Health care personnel is addressed in Chapter 9. Particular emphasis is given to physicians who represent perhaps the most critical of the personnel resources in terms of decision making and policy development. Chapter 10 describes the nation's pharmaceutical industry, which is increasingly playing a critical role in providing therapeutic alternatives and solutions to the diseases faced by our nation, and the role of technology.

Part 3 assesses how we pay for, manage, control, and evaluate the nation's health care system. Chapter 11 focuses on insurance and reimburse-ment mechanisms, which in effect are the organizing force and overall control mechanism for the system itself. Chapter 12 describes the role of specific managed care mechanisms and organizations in effecting change and managing resources in the nation's health care system. Chapter 13 examines other regulatory and planning mechanisms that have been utilized in the past and some potential regulatory mechanisms for the future. Chapter 14, examines how we measure and assess the quality of care provided. Finally, Chapter 15 examines national health policy and politics and its effect on how the health care system has evolved and its potential effect in the future.

CONCLUDING COMMENTS

As health care and medicine have become increasingly complicated, so, too, have the organization and structure of the nation's health care system. It is important for everyone involved in the health care field to understand these complexities and interrelationships. It is not a bad idea for consumers, as well, to gain a better perspective on the system that they depend on for their lives and well-being. It is to these ends that this book is dedicated as an educational resource for anyone interested in a relatively uncomplicated description of a complicated system, a system that is increasingly dominating our national thoughts, economy, and concerns.

Stephen J. Williams
San Diego, California

Acknowledgments

Unless otherwise indicated, data tables are derived from:

>National Center for Health Statistics
>Health, United States, 2003
>Hyattsville, Maryland: Public Health
>   Service, 2003

At press time, the 2004 edition of this terrific data resource was being released by the federal government. It is available on the Internet at: http://www.cdc.gov/nchs/hus.htm

Annual updates with new data are published by the National Center for Health Statistics.

Number totals in some tables are subject to rounding and reporting error. Sometimes similar data are presented from different sources, resulting in minor discrepancies. Debbie Doan greatly assisted in the preparation of the manuscript. The publishing team of Thomson Delmar Learning turned the manuscript into a finely produced textbook. Anonymous reviewers provided many valuable suggestions.

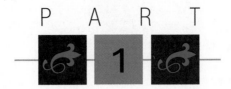

An Overview of Health Care in the United States

This part of the book starts the discussion with a look at the big picture. A statistical and descriptive overview of the nation's health care system is presented in text and tables.

CHAPTER 1

The Big Picture

Chapter Objectives

1. To present an overview of the health care system.
2. To present national health care expenditures by category.

Our nation's health care system is one of its largest and most important economic activities. The health care system, with its component parts, consumes more than $1.5 trillion in gross domestic product (GDP) annually; employs approximately 13 million individuals; contributes to our nation's overall well-being and productivity and to our longevity and quality of life; and serves as a significant focal point for our social, economic, and political systems.

The delivery of health services in this country pervades our daily life and challenges us constantly with complex issues and concerns, both individually and collectively. The demands of ensuring the health and well-being of more than 295 million Americans requires a constant national effort directed at protecting our health and intervening to address illness and injury. Health care services are provided throughout the nation on a 24-hour basis, and are constantly ready to respond to the needs of our population. At the same time, they present numerous challenges totally dissimilar from those found in most other sectors of the economy.

The overarching objective of the nation's health care system is to improve the quality and length of life for our citizens. These achievements are measurable in terms of number of years of life, measures of disability such as work days lost, and other indicators of our health and well-being. Achieving this complex goal requires an expensive and complex national effort. The design and operation of the nation's health care system must respond to an immense array of amazingly intricate needs on the part of the population. The examination of this complex system is the subject of this book, with a particular focus on the core themes of access to health care, paying for services, decision making within the system, and measuring the function of the health care system and its component parts. In spite of our immense efforts in operating the nation's health care system, however, many people, perhaps 40 million, still lack access to health care because of inadequate or absent health insurance or other financial resources. The challenges we face are immense and seem to grow each day, but our responses often have been tremendously successful and dramatic as well.

The beginning chapters of this book are designed to provide a framework for exploring and understanding the complex nature of health care services in the United States. The entire structure of this book is based on the premise that an analytical, population-based perspective is essential to comprehend fully the many complexities of the health care environment.

No part of our economy is as vital to our individual and national well-being as health care. Yet this sector may be the least understood and most controversial aspect of our nation's economy. Understanding these challenges and gaining an appreciation for the complex nature of the organization, financing, and regulation of health care services are absolutely essential for any participant in the system.

As we move into the middle of the first decade of the twenty-first century, many of the fundamental themes and concerns that we have heard during the past 100 years regarding the nation's health care system continue to roil our collective thinking. The onrush of increasingly sophisticated technology does not seem to be matched by an equal degree of advancement in medical services delivery. Concerns about access, costs, assessment and evaluation, quality, and planning are still heard constantly. Indeed, the continuing evolution of health care in the United States follows a long-standing pattern of technical progress and complex delivery issues, which ultimately never seem to be adequately addressed to meet our economic, social, political, and equity needs. But our increasing ability to intervene in the progression of disease, or to avert the occurrence of disease, suggests that the payoff from a more efficient and effective delivery system will be more substantial than ever before in our nation's history.

HISTORICAL EVOLUTION

The health care system has progressed through numerous phases of change and challenge over the centuries since the founding of the nation. Prior to the beginning of the twentieth century, the health care system faced the challenges of a predominance of acute infectious diseases, epidemics, and frequently unhealthy work and living environments for our nation's population. Little technological capability was available to provide a response by the nation's primordial health care system. Individuals with serious diseases, unless the disease was self-limiting, frequently succumbed to their illnesses. A sturdy genetic composition, in retrospect, was essential for survival.

Although many individuals did live to a ripe old age, at least in the context of the 1700s and 1800s, high rates of mortality were experienced by infants and children, and other causes of mortality took their toll as well on the remainder of the population. The nation's health care system itself was relatively unorganized and oriented primarily toward the provision of care by solo practice physicians. Some indigent care was made available through the hospitals, almshouses, and other institutional providers at the time. More detailed historical information regarding each of the settings in which care is provided is contained in the chapters that follow.

From the early part of the twentieth century until World War II, particularly at the conclusion of the war, the delivery of health services became slightly more structured and began to embrace a scientific basis for the practice of medicine. Particularly in the early part of the twentieth century, medical education became revolutionized and a more analytical approach to providing care was instituted. This period still represented a very tentative step toward the application of modern technology, but formed the origins of today's much more advanced delivery system. The technological approach and more formal organization of services we see today evolved from these earlier roots.

A key turning point in the history of the nation's approach to health and social services during this era was the passage of legislation comprising the New Deal of President Franklin D. Roosevelt. The establishment of the nation's Social Security system and a dramatic redefinition of the role of government in assisting its citizenry were especially notable in this period. These political, economic, and philosophical changes eventually formed the basis for much more extensive and direct government intervention in the nation's health care system during the 1960s with the passage of President Lyndon B. Johnson's Great Society legislation.

The first phase of the era of truly modern medicine can be traced back to the immediate post-World War II period. The expansion of technology; the passage of extensive federal legislation leading to government involvement in health care services; increasing structural reorganization of the health care system through both public and private avenues; and dramatic changes in the economic, political, and ethical environments for health care can all be traced back to this time.

From the end of World War II until approximately the middle to late 1980s, the nation's health care system expanded dramatically, bringing to bear an increasing array of technological innovations and therapeutic interventions. Government involvement in health services directly and indirectly expanded. Increasing emphasis on chronic diseases, such as heart disease, cancer, and stroke, established new and critical priorities for health care delivery and for national expenditures. Increasingly, health care gained national attention as a source of information for public consumption, for political consideration, and for national debate.

The most recent phase of development in the nation's health care system, again dating approximately from the late 1980s to the present and projected into the future, is characterized by increasing structure, monitoring, and evaluation of the nation's health care system; expansive new technologies; increasing financial pressures and political concerns; and much greater public awareness and debate regarding health care issues. This current phase of development in the nation's health care system has at least partially been triggered by dramatic new advances in biomedical knowledge resulting from investment in basic research.

The delivery of health services is based on the increasing knowledge of human biology at the molecular level and has triggered great advances in diagnosis and treatment throughout all aspects of somatic and mental health. Yet these advances are only in their early stages and promise even more dramatic and fundamental changes for future care. Because changes such as these so dramatically impact the delivery of health care services we can also anticipate continued turbulence, reorganization, and rediscovery in the mechanisms through which we provide health care services to our nation's population. At the same time, the increasing cost of services and complex ethical and moral issues have forced numerous access, financing, and delivery concerns to the front of our national agenda.

In addition, many issues that we have failed to address adequately over the past 100 years are still on our plate. These include providing services to uninsured and underinsured people, defining national priorities and rationing, accessing new technologies and introducing them in an appropriate way, and properly evaluating the quality and appropriateness of the care that is provided.

The current phase of health care services is also characterized by the increasing delivery of services through proprietary or for-profit channels; consolidation of systems of services through numerous for-profit, not-for-profit, and governmental entities; and a constant and challenging reassessment of the structure, organization, and operation of all aspects of the nation's health care delivery system.

The challenges today are greater than ever before, yet so are the opportunities. Never in our history have we faced as many complex organizational and economic issues with regard to structuring health care delivery, yet never before have we

had such great opportunities to substantially improve the health of our nation's population. While this current phase of development is the most challenging, it is also the most exciting and the one that holds the greatest promise for the future.

NATIONAL HEALTH EXPENDITURES

Never in the history of the world has any major nation spent as much of its national financial resources on health care as does the United States currently. Whether measured as a percentage of total GDP, the total of all goods and services produced in the country, or on a per capita or total dollar basis, the United States spends far more than any other country in the world for health care services, and has done so for quite some time.

Although the principal focus of this book is on health care services in the United States, occasional reference to international perspectives is valuable in placing issues of health care delivery in the United States in a broader perspective. Each and every country in the world is unique in many ways, and cross-national comparisons are often difficult and even inappropriate. Such comparisons, however, often do provide an opportunity to highlight issues that we face in a context that is not otherwise available. Understanding the nature of these international differences and then assessing why the United States appears to have unique or different concerns with regard to health care is an excellent exercise for students when they think about our own nation's health care system. At the same time, recognizing the many advantages that we have in this nation compared to most other countries is useful in understanding our own good fortune.

Table 1.1 presents a brief international perspective on health care expenditures for the United States and selected other countries. As discussed later in this book, in spite of such dramatic national expenditures allocated to health care services, our longevity is far from the best of any

Table 1.1. Total Health Expenditures as a Percentage of Gross Domestic Product and Per Capita Health Expenditures in Dollars: Selected Countries and Years 1960–2000

Country	1960	1980	2000
Health expenditures as a percentage of gross domestic product			
Australia	4.3	7.0	8.3
Canada	5.4	7.1	9.1
France	—	—	9.5
Germany	4.8	8.8	10.6
Greece	—	6.6	8.3
Italy	3.6	—	8.1
Japan	3.0	6.4	7.8
Korea	—	—	5.9
Mexico	—	—	5.4
Switzerland	4.9	7.6	10.7
United Kingdom	3.9	5.6	7.3
United States	5.1	8.8	13.3
Per capita health expenditures			
Australia	$87	$658	$2,211
Canada	109	710	2,535
France	—	—	2,349
Germany	90	824	2,748
Greece	—	348	1,399
Italy	48	—	2,032
Japan	26	522	2,012
Korea	—	—	893
Mexico	—	—	490
Switzerland	136	881	3,222
United Kingdom	74	444	1,763
United States	143	1,067	4,672

country in the world. However, we have faced more complex challenges than many other countries, and our heterogeneous population presents a very complex palate of health care problems and challenges. Incredibly, health care expenditures in the United States now (in 2005) exceed 14 percent of GDP, more than twice that for the United

Kingdom and more than those of any other country in the world as well. Parenthetically, most developing countries spend a relatively small percentage of GDP on health care services by allocating such expenditures to public health services and, where feasible, to both public and private delivery of care.

The percentage of our nation's GDP allocated to health care has been increasing dramatically over the years and particularly since the 1960s. Prior to the explosion of government spending, particularly in the 1960s, our expenditures for health care were not dramatically greater than those of many other countries, such as Canada. While expenditures in virtually all countries have increased since 1960, those for the United States have increased at a greater rate and to a more dramatic level than any other country in the world.

On a per capita expenditure basis, the United States spends more than $4,000 for every man, woman, and child on average, per year, for health care services. Total expenditures exceed $1.5 trillion per year and, most telling, the percentage of all our economic activity allocated to health care has continued to increase—now exceeding approximately 14 percent.

As the percentage of gross domestic product allocated to health care services increases, expenditures for other sectors have to decrease. The pie can add only to 100 percent. Thus, the increasing demands for health care mean sacrifices for other sectors of the economy as dollars are shifted to the health care arena. This shift represents a significant collective national decision as to the allocation of our national resources. These choices are made collectively, through government, and individually, through personal spending decisions.

Table 1.2 provides the elaboration of national health expenditures for the United States for selected years. Again, the growth of spending in absolute dollars and percentage of GDP and in per capita expenditures is evident and dramatic. Table 1.2 also provides ample evidence of the increasing role of government in national health expenditures

Table 1.2. GDP, National Health Expenditures, and Federal, State, and Local Government Health Expenditures: United States, Selected Years

| | | National Health Expenditures | | | Federal Government Expenditures | State and Local Government Expenditures |
Year	GDP in Billions	Amount in Billions	Percentage of GDP	Amount per Capita	Amount in Billions	Amount in Billions
1960	$527	$26.9	5.1	$141	$2.9	$3.7
1970	1,036	73.2	7.1	341	17.8	9.9
1980	2,784	247.3	8.9	1,052	72.0	32.8
1990	5,744	699.5	12.2	2,691	195.8	88.5
2001	10,082	1,424.5	14.1	5,035	454.8	191.8

since the passage of a variety of legislative initiatives during the Great Society of President Lyndon B. Johnson.

Although the federal government used to be a relatively minor, but not insignificant, player in providing funding for health care–related services, that has changed dramatically with federal, state, and local governments now representing major sources of expenditures for health care. These sources include the Medicare and Medicaid programs.

Federal expenditures for health care services have exploded under Medicare, Medicaid, and other governmental programs. State and local expenditures, which were always important, have also increased, particularly with the state portion of funding for the Medicaid program for medically indigent individuals. These governmental programs are further defined and explained in later chapters of this book, but at this point, suffice it to say that they are major drivers in the increase in health care costs and national political priorities.

The end of the twentieth century and the initial years of the twenty-first century were marked by an economic business cycle that went from high growth into recession followed by relatively sluggish economic recovery. These trends, combined with the Bush administration tax cuts and the fiscal pressures from the War on Terrorism, resulted in substantially increased pressure on state and local government funding of health care services, particularly for the Medicaid program. State government receipts from various forms of taxation combined with a slowing economic environment meant that competition for money among such key state and local services as education, law enforcement, fire protection, and health care was substantially increased, while demands for health and social and welfare services also were increasing with rising unemployment. By early 2005, the situation had improved a lot.

This recent period of economic stress highlights the fragile nature of funding for health care in the United States, particularly for services to meet the needs of the elderly and those with limited financial resources. The cost of providing such services is so high, and the numbers of individuals seeking to qualify for these benefits is so great, that many states face a serious fiscal crisis on a relatively regular basis. These financial pressures are unlikely to abate any time soon. The fierce debate in the U.S. Congress over revisions to the Medicare program, including the addition of an outpatient pharmacy benefit, further illustrates these issues.

In examining health care expenditures, it is vital to keep in mind that all dollars spent on health care emanate from the same source; that is, the individual citizens of the nation. Dollars spent by federal, state, and local government entities are collected from the citizens through taxation, fees, and deficit spending. Dollars expended by employers are collected from consumers as corporations include health care costs in the price of goods and services produced. For example, when you purchase a domestically produced automobile, perhaps $1,000 or more of the purchase price of that vehicle is utilized to pay for health care benefits for employees and retirees of the automotive manufacturers and their suppliers.

In recent years, with the general decline in economic growth combined with competitive international market pressures, many employers have been substantially cutting back, or even eliminating, retiree health care benefits. Retirees are facing huge increases in their costs of obtaining health care coverage. The situation is particularly acute for individuals who are not yet old enough to qualify for the federal Medicare program and who have retired under the assumption that their employer-sponsored health care benefits will continue at least until they qualify for Medicare. In addition, many companies are reducing or even dropping health care benefits.

Since our nation is in uncharted territory with regard to total expenditures and the percentage of GDP allocated to health care services, it is very difficult to assess what limits we may face in the future. We have certainly heard the call for cost containment over the years, yet health care expenditures continue to increase. When and how any absolute limits will be reached is unknown at the present time. Whether health care services can continue to claim a larger and larger share of gross domestic product at the expense of other sectors of the economy within the context of the nation's political system is uncertain. As pressures continue to build, new efforts to limit costs through basic structural change, such as managed care providers, will be necessary. More efficient use of resources and lower-cost technologies are also absolutely essential for the future. Following how the nation responds to all of these political, economic, and social pressures and the ramifications for our health and well-being will be an essential theme in future years.

Government's Role in Health Care Spending

Table 1.3 illustrates the increasing involvement of governments in the financing of health care services. Government spending on health care and government spending as a percentage of total national health care costs have increased substantially over time. The most significant increases have occurred since the passage of Medicare and Medicaid and other social legislation in the middle 1960s.

Government spending includes federal government expenditures, particularly for the Medicare program and the federal share of the Medicaid program, as well as a variety of other activities, including the National Institutes of Health, the Public Health Service, the Indian Health Service, and the Veterans Administration. State and local government spending, which has increased substantially as well, includes the state share of Medicaid expenditures as well as a wide range of local services.

Expenditure Categories

National health expenditures are allocated to a wide range of activities. Table 1.4 presents, for various years, the specific categories of expenditures included in the overall national health care bill.

Historically, hospital-related costs have accounted for approximately 30 to 40 percent of total health care expenditures. Even with the increasing prominence of other sectors of the health care industry, the hospital still accounts for nearly 40 percent of all health care dollars. Physician professional services expenditures have accounted for approximately 18 to 20 percent of the health care bill and have remained fairly stable over time.

Table 1.3. National Health Expenditures According to Source of Funds: United States, Selected Years

	All Health Expenditures in Billions	Private Funds		Public Funds	
Year		Amount in Billions	Percentage of Total	Amount in Billions	Percentage of Total
1940	$4.0	$3.2	79.7	$0.8	20.3
1950	12.7	9.2	72.8	3.4	27.2
1960	27.1	20.5	75.5	6.7	24.5
1970	74.4	46.7	62.8	27.7	37.2
1980	250.1	145.0	58.0	105.2	42.0
1990	699.5	415.1	59.3	284.4	40.7
2001	1,424.5	777.9	54.6	646.7	45.4

Substantial increases in the share of the health care pie allocated to long-term care services and to a number of smaller sectors have occurred. The share spent on pharmaceuticals and related items has actually declined. Administration, research, and construction account for relatively modest percentages of the health care dollar.

It should be noted that, in Table 1.4, personal health services are defined as those involving the direct delivery of clinical services. Nonpersonal expenditures are those allocated to governmental prevention programs, research, construction, and other population-based activities.

In the future, the share of the health care dollar allocated to home health care, long-term care, and drugs and pharmaceuticals is likely to increase. Increasing utilization of noninstitutionally based care such as ambulatory surgery, home health, pharmaceutical therapies provided outside of the hospital, and various technological innovations should further shift the focus from hospital inpatient care to other settings.

Over a long period of time, but particularly in the past few years, substantial attention has been directed toward the increasing costs of pharmaceutical products. Many insurance plans require a significant payment on the part of enrollees to help pay for the cost of pharmaceuticals. The federal Medicare program historically has not covered most outpatient pharmaceutical products at all. Biomedical research over the past 25 years has yielded a significant pipeline of new products to treat a wide variety of illnesses. The costs of developing these products and their marketing, distribution, and related administrative costs are bundled into the pricing of pharmaceutical products. As a result, pharmaceutical costs, particularly those related to prescription drugs, have escalated dramatically in terms of both individual product pricing and total national expenditures. There is tremendous political pressure to address the increased costs of this sector of the health care system. In attempting to assign blame for health care cost increases, and in recognizing the historically high degree of profitability of pharmaceutical product companies, political and economic pressure has been brought to bear on these firms. Efforts are being directed toward reducing the use of costly products when less expensive alternatives exist, reducing product pricing, importation of products from outside the country, and other attempts to contain cost increases in the prescription drug marketplace.

The allocation of health care dollars by payer category is illustrated further in Table 1.5. Changes in the share paid by individuals out of their own pockets as well as by private health

Table 1.4. National Health Expenditures, Average Annual Percentage Change, and Percentage Distribution, According to Type of Expenditure: United States, Selected Years 1960–2001

Type of Expenditure	1960	1980	2000	2001	2001
					Amount in billions
	Percent distribution				
National health expenditures	100.0	100.0	100.0	100.0	$1,424.5
Health services and supplies	93.6	95.0	96.4	96.4	1,372.6
Personal health care	87.6	87.3	86.8	86.8	1,236.4
Hospital care	34.4	41.3	31.8	31.7	451.2
Professional services	31.3	27.4	32.4	32.5	462.4
Physician and clinical services	20.1	19.2	22.0	22.0	313.6
Other professional services	1.5	1.5	3.0	3.0	42.3
Dental services	7.4	5.4	4.6	4.6	65.6
Other personal health care	2.4	1.3	2.8	2.9	40.9
Nursing home and home health	3.4	8.2	9.6	9.3	132.1
Home health care	0.2	1.0	2.4	2.3	33.2
Nursing home care	3.2	7.2	7.2	6.9	98.9
Retail outlet sales of medical products	18.6	10.5	13.0	13.4	190.7
Prescription drugs	10.0	4.9	9.3	9.9	140.6
Other medical products	8.5	5.6	3.7	3.5	50.1
Government administration and net cost of private health insurance	4.5	4.9	6.2	6.3	89.7
Government public health activities	1.5	2.7	3.4	3.3	46.4
Investment	6.4	5.0	3.6	3.6	52.0
Research (government)	2.6	2.2	2.2	2.3	32.8
Construction	3.8	2.8	1.4	1.3	19.2

insurance and by government are presented in this table.

Interestingly, individuals still pay a significant portion of all health care dollars as out-of-pocket expenses unreimbursed by any third party and not paid for by government. Of course, it must be kept in mind that individuals actually pay all health care costs, since government expenditures are paid through taxation and debt financing, while the costs of employer-sponsored health care benefits are included in the pricing of goods and services.

CHALLENGES FOR THE FUTURE

The organization and structure of the nation's health care system are driven, at least in part, by the underlying need and demand for health care. These forces are, in turn, a function of demographic factors, patterns of disease and illness, changing perceptions of disease, and technological capabilities. The dynamics of health care services in the United States are constantly changing as a result of these forces and of var-

Table 1.5. Personal Health Care Expenditures and Percentage Distribution, According to Source of Funds: United States, Selected Years

| | | | | | | | Government | | |
Year	Total in Billions	Per Capita	All Sources	Out-of-Pocket Payments	Private Health Insurance	Other Private Funds	Total	Federal	State and Local
				Percent distribution					
1950	10.9	70	100.0	65.5	9.1	2.9	22.4	10.4	12.0
1970	64.9	302	100.0	39.5	23.4	2.6	34.6	22.6	12.0
1990	614.7	2,364	100.0	23.5	33.6	3.5	39.4	28.9	10.5
2001	1,236.4	4,370	100.0	16.6	35.4	4.6	43.4	32.9	10.6

ious financial and political issues. Providers, consumers, payers, and policymakers are constantly vying for power and authority within the system. And, unlike many other aspects of our economy, health care is fundamental to our very survivability.

The rate of change in the health care system, especially with regard to politics, economics, and technology, is also accelerating. Biomedical research is leading to rapid change as scientific discoveries are more quickly translated into clinical practice.

The overwhelming financial burden of providing health care services to all of our citizens becomes more complex and critical as the dollars involved become larger and represent a greater percentage of our GDP. The demographic forces, particularly those associated with an aging population, also accelerate the political pressures on policymakers and on government officials to come to grips with such truly difficult problems as providing care for uninsured and underinsured individuals, and allocating scarce resources within the system.

The stakes are exceedingly high in health care, and the decision making is highly complex, dependent on numerous factors that themselves involve massive political, economic, and social considerations. The answers are not clear-cut. Competing demands from all sectors of our society

place great strain on our ability to address the many complexities of health care rationally.

Ultimately, as a nation we must come to grips with the many challenges of the health care system. We must collectively decide such complex issues as the extent to which government at its various levels will be involved in the delivery or financing of health care services. We must determine the role of the consumer, including his or her responsibility for living a healthy lifestyle to reduce reliance on health services. Our nation must address how to provide care and finance services for individuals who lack adequate insurance or coverage under social programs.

We must determine how technology will be diffused throughout the system, how it will be evaluated, and when it will be made available to all citizens. We must make the ultimate trade-offs as to how much of our national resources will be allocated to health care, as opposed to other economic activities. And, ultimately, we must decide how to provide care in the most effective and efficient manner possible.

Our nation has experienced considerable trauma in the evolution of health services since its founding. We have many successes and some significant failures on our scorecard. In international comparisons, we spend more than any nation in the history of mankind on health care, both in absolute dollars and as a percentage of GDP. But

we also have the most sophisticated and richly sup-
plied system on the planet today.

Our tremendous capabilities are the envy of the
world, and they certainly justify much of the
resources that we have invested. And the social and
political difficulties that we have experienced have
helped ensure the health of our nation.

As we face the future we can look back on a
difficult but ultimately progressive past. We do
have a solid platform from which to move forward from here. In spite of the many problems
that we face, the opportunities are equally great.
It is the role of all who are involved in the health

care system to push forward toward greater efficiency and quality in assuring health care for all
Americans.

STUDY QUESTIONS

1. What is the economic scope of the nation's
   health care system in terms of dollar expenditures and the use of those dollars?
2. The United States spends more than any other
   developed country on health care services.
   Why is that?
3. Who really pays for health care and how?

CHAPTER 2

The Underlying Basis for Health Services Utilization

Chapter Objectives

1. To examine national social and economic trends as they pertain to health care needs.
2. To examine national trends in fertility and mortality.
3. To describe national disease patterns.
4. To determine the advantages of preventive services.

This chapter examines the social, demographic, psychological, and sociological bases for the need for health care services in the United States. Extensive emphasis is placed on examining available analytical data that reflect patterns of population, behavior, social demographic trends, and other analytical perspectives on the characteristics of our population and its need for health care services. Only through analyzing and understanding the underlying measurable and quantitative indicators of the characteristics of the population can we objectively and clinically assess our current needs, limitations, and challenges.

Although an examination of quantitative data may seem tedious, such an analytical approach allows us to make decisions and formulate recommendations based on a more solid factual foundation than simply guessing or observing the behavior of a few individuals. This analytical approach to assessing and understanding the health care system is essential for rational long-term decision making in spite of the many emotional, political, and social aspects that come into play when people utilize health care services.

THE BIOLOGICAL BASIS FOR HEALTH SERVICES UTILIZATION

Fundamentally, utilization of health care services is a function of underlying biological processes and individual consumer and professional responses to perceptions of those processes. Our knowledge of disease, and the underlying pathophysiology of the human body, has changed dramatically over the past 50 years. Medical education and practice have increasingly focused on the molecular basis for disease and illness, reflecting a much greater depth of understanding of biological processes. Dramatic changes in imaging, measurement of biological variables, and truly fundamental improvement in available interventions have radically altered the practice of medicine. These changes have brought about equally dramatic changes in the health care delivery system and continuing needs to reassess our fundamental approaches to the organization of health care in the United States.

At the same time these changes have coincided with enhanced public perceptions and expectations, creating tremendous pressures on those who organize and provide services. Expensive new technologies for diagnosis and intervention, while delivering on promises for reduction in morbidity and mortality, have also raised fundamental questions about access, costs, and appropriateness of outcomes. As longevity increases, these issues will continue to gain in importance in the continuing debate regarding providing comprehensive services to all Americans.

It is important to differentiate an individual's perception of illness and disease from that of a health care professional. Frequently, individuals' perceptions are not consistent with those resulting from professional evaluation. Disease is characterized as specific signs and symptoms and measures and evaluations that reflect various pathophysiologic processes. An individual's perception of illness may not fit a professional's evaluation of disease.

The predominant diseases of a population can change over time and across countries. New diseases are discovered frequently. National priorities for research and intervention based on the prevalence of various disease categories entail tremendous political and economic considerations such that research expenditures and intervention efforts may not be totally consistent with disease patterns for a particular country.

Even in the face of tremendous biomedical progress and much greater understanding of the basic science of biology there is increased interest in our country in alternative approaches to providing care. The Federal National Institutes of Health has created an office for further investigation of alternative medicine approaches, and many individuals seek such care from time to time. Such alternative medicine approaches as acupuncture, herbal medicine, dietary supplementation, and other healing methods are gaining popularity, even in some medical circles. These approaches challenge the delivery system's focus on traditional medicine for diagnosis and intervention. It seems somewhat ironic that in an era of greatly enhanced scientific knowledge we recognize the potential contributions of approaches that have been available for many centuries, and that are based on a variety of concepts developed on a more evolutionary and practical basis.

THE NEED FOR HEALTH CARE SERVICES

Generally speaking, the need, demand, and actual utilization of health care services are conceptualized separately in analyzing patient behavior in the health care system. Need is usually defined as professionally assessed or clinically identifiable justification for the use of health care services. For example, a physician evaluating a patient's complaints would determine the clinical basis for a need for additional services, such as through clinical testing.

The demand for health care services is defined, particularly by health economists, as patient care-seeking behavior, which translates into attempts to obtain health care services. These attempts may or may not be successful depending on a patient's access to health care, considering such factors as the availability of services, the financial ability of the patient to obtain care, and physical access.

Need and demand for health care may not be equal. For example, individuals may seek care for services that a clinician feels are not necessary. Conversely, a clinician may recommend care that the patient decides against seeking.

When translated into actual consumption of care, the need and demand for health services yield what is termed use or utilization. Utilization, in turn, is measured by such variables as hospital days per thousand population or physician office visits per person.

Care-seeking behavior, particularly demand for health services, is often also a function of numerous sociodemographic characteristics of patients. Research by health care sociologists has demonstrated differences in care-seeking behavior based on ethnic group and other social characteristics.

Research by psychologists and others demonstrates the effect of attitudes on care-seeking behavior. For example, individuals who believe that health care services are likely to help them are more likely to seek care than those who are skeptical of medical practice.

Attitudes can play a very significant role in determining who seeks health care services and under what conditions. Attitudes can also impact clinical outcomes, probably by affecting the immune system. Thus, understanding the various characteristics of a population is important in planning for the potential use of health services, as well as for removing physical, psychological, and emotional barriers to care.

THE DEMOGRAPHIC ORIGINS OF HEALTH SERVICES UTILIZATION

Approximately 15 to 20 percent of the increase in health care costs in the United States over the past 30 years is attributable to increases in the size of the country's population and changes in the distribution of population by age group. Table 2.1 illustrates the growth of the resident population of the United States by age category.

The increasing size of the population means a greater need for health care resources. Thus, some increases in the dollar cost of health care are inherently unavoidable with a growing population. However, the interplay between population growth, economic growth, and the components of health care costs, such as technology and cost inflation, are extremely complex; numerous changes in many other factors have occurred along with the increase in the country's population.

Second, changes in the demographic age structure of the population, such as those that have occurred over the past 40-plus years, also change the nature of the need and demand for health care services. The nation's population has been aging, with an increasing proportion of the population reaching older ages, particularly 65 years and above. As the population ages, and as a greater proportion of people are in the older age groups, the demand and need for health care increases, since people 65 years of age and older on average utilize 50 to 100 percent more health care services per capita than the younger population.

The relationship between utilization and age for specific health care services is discussed in more detail later in this book. It is important here to point out that, with both an increase in the absolute numbers of individuals 65 years of age and older and with a greater proportion of the population falling into the older age groups, demand for health care services, particularly for more expensive institutional services, will tend to increase.

The population of the United States is likely to continue to increase as a result of both the natural rate of increase, that is, the excess of births over deaths, and net in-migration, well into the twenty-first century. In addition, the population of the country on average is continuing to age, with a still greater percentage of the population likely to fall into elderly age groups during the first two decades of the twenty-first century.

These demographic trends by themselves suggest an increasing need for health care services. Add in technological advances and other factors germane to the older age groups, and the effect is exacerbated.

Thus, demographic trends are of immense importance in understanding the need and demand for health care and patterns of utilization. Furthermore, geographic differences in the demographic structure of populations mean that differences can occur across various localities throughout the country. For example, states such as Florida, with a disproportionately large percentage of their populations in the older age groups, will experience even greater demand for health care services because of these demographic factors.

Of course, these demographic trends change over time and interact with health care needs and use in many different ways. For example, the proportion of individuals migrating into the United States who are younger and healthier would represent a less significant current demand for health

Table 2.1. Resident Population, by Age: United States, Selected Years

	Total Resident Population	Under 1 Year	1–4 Years	5–14 Years	15–24 Years	25–34 Years	35–44 Years	45–54 Years	55–64 Years	65–74 Years	75–84 Years	85 Years and Older
					Number in thousands							
1950	150,697	3,147	13,017	24,319	22,098	23,759	21,450	17,343	13,370	8,340	3,278	577
1960	179,323	4,112	16,209	35,465	24,020	22,818	24,081	20,485	15,572	10,997	4,633	929
1970	203,212	3,485	13,669	40,746	35,441	24,907	23,088	23,220	18,590	12,435	6,119	1,511
1980	222,546	3,534	12,815	34,942	42,487	37,082	25,635	22,800	21,703	15,581	7,729	2,240
1990	248,710	3,946	14,812	35,095	37,013	43,161	37,435	25,057	21,113	18,045	10,012	3,021
2001	284,797	4,034	15,336	41,065	39,948	39,607	45,019	39,188	25,309	18,313	12,574	4,404

care services than an older immigrant population, but in the longer term would imply a significant eventual increase in health care service utilization as these individuals reach the older ages. A young immigrant population might have a relatively high fertility rate, leading to increased use of reproductive and pediatric services. Other characteristics of a migratory population such as differences in proportion of males versus females might also likewise impact utilization of services. Social demographic characteristics are also important. An immigrant who is well skilled and able to obtain employment, perhaps with health care benefits, would be less of a social burden to state and local governments in particular than would be a less skilled and likely uninsured or underinsured person. Demographic trends are complicated and require thoughtful analysis and longer-term projections to fully understand their implications for the nation's health care industry. Of course, we must all keep in mind that more than 99 percent of all Americans are here as a result of immigration into the country. Demand for health care services in the absence of migration would be quite modest.

FERTILITY AND HEALTH SERVICES

The size of the domestic population is obviously determined in part by the natural increase in population. The natural increase in population, as noted previously, is the excess of births over deaths. The greater the number of births, the greater the demand for obstetrical and pediatric care. Of course, the number of births affects numerous social, economic, and financial factors, such as the demand for social services such as education, health care, and welfare. The politics and economic and social structures of a population are also dependent on the proportion of the population that is comprised of children and young adults. These people generally do not contribute to economic productivity but rather represent a dependency burden on the

working population as do older, retired people. Thus, birth rate trends, and the absolute numbers of births, have a direct relationship to many aspects of a society, including health care.

Table 2.2 presents the number of births and birth rates for the U.S. population over time. Birth rates are presented for specific age groups within the population. The changes in the distribution of births, and relative birth rates for each age group, are evident in this table for selected years.

The Great Depression led to a decline in fertility but, at the end of World War II, birth rates exploded with the baby boom. This was followed by a long decline in fertility rates beginning in the mid–1950s and continuing through the 1960s. Increasing labor force participation by women was a major cause of this decline.

At the present time, the nation is experiencing about four million births per year with relatively greater numbers of births in the very young ages and moderately greater numbers in the somewhat older ages. Remarkably, of the four million births per year, over one million are to unmarried women, a much greater percentage than was experienced in earlier years (Table 2.3). Recently, there has been a decline in births to teen and unmarried mothers in the United States.

Dramatic changes in the social structure of the nation that are related to fertility patterns include substantially fewer numbers of individuals in traditional marriages, with more than one million divorces per year and approximately one million children affected by divorce annually. Divorce tends to create lower standards of living for the divorced wife and for the children. Health insurance, psychological problems, and other ramifications of divorce are also increasingly prevalent in our society.

In recent years, the rate of divorce has stabilized somewhat. Still, divorce inflicts tremendous adverse costs on our society. Other related social trends such as increased cohabitation, later age at first marriage, and economic pressures on existing marriages also impact the social structure and

Table 2.2. Live Births, Crude Birth Rates, and Birth Rates by Age of Mother: United States, Selected Years

| | Live Births | Fertility Rate | Crude Birth Rate | Age of Mother | | | | | | | | |
				10–14 Years	15–17 Years	18–19 Years	20–24 Years	25–29 Years	30–34 Years	35–39 Years	40–44 Years	45–54 Years
				Live Births per 1,000 women								
1950	3,632,000	106.2	24.1	1.0	40.7	132.7	196.6	166.1	103.7	52.9	15.1	1.2
1960	4,257,850	118.0	23.7	0.8	43.9	166.7	258.1	197.4	112.7	56.2	15.5	0.9
1970	3,731,386	87.9	18.4	1.2	38.8	114.7	167.8	145.1	73.3	31.7	8.1	0.5
1980	3,612,258	68.4	15.9	1.1	32.5	82.1	115.1	112.9	61.9	19.8	3.9	0.2
1990	4,153,212	70.9	16.7	1.4	37.5	88.6	116.5	120.2	80.8	31.7	5.5	0.2
2001	4,025,933	65.3	14.1	0.8	24.7	76.1	106.2	113.4	91.9	40.6	8.1	0.5

eventually the health status and health care behaviors of our population. Countervailing trends, such as relatively popular remarriage, increasing home ownership, and generally improved living standards, probably partially offset the negative consequences of adverse social and behavioral patterns. The interplay of these many highly complex economic and sociological factors in our society is extremely difficult to analyze and to project long term into the future, particularly as they pertain to the use of health care services. Health care policymakers and analysts must constantly monitor and assess these changing trends.

Mortality Patterns and Health Care Services

As is the case for fertility, mortality patterns have a great influence on health care utilization. Causes of morbidity and mortality affect the types of health care services that people use, and trends in mortality affect how long people live and how much health care they consume over their lifetimes. Mortality is also an outcome measure of the effectiveness of the health care system, although many other factors, particularly those associated with lifestyle, economic well-being, and individual genetic composition greatly influence life expectancy.

From an international perspective, life expectancy comparisons across countries provide some insight into the relative experiences of individuals in different geographic locations and in different social and political environments. Table 2.4 presents international life expectancy data for selected countries.

Data are presented separately for males and females owing to the highly significant difference in

Table 2.3. Nonmarital Childbearing: United States, 1970–2001

Race of Mother	1970	1985	2001
	Percentage of live births to unmarried mothers		
All races	10.7	22.0	33.5
White	5.5	14.7	27.7
Black or African American	37.5	61.2	68.4
American Indian or Alaska Native	22.4	46.8	59.7
Asian or Pacific Islander	—	9.5	14.9
Hispanic or Latino	—	29.5	42.5
	Number of live births, in thousands		
Live births to unmarried mothers	399	828	1,349

longevity by sex. Although the underlying social and biological factors associated with this differential have not been completely elucidated, numerous factors have been identified, at least partially, to explain them. These factors include differences associated with coronary artery disease, possibly attributable to hormonal differences; differences in lifestyles; risk factors associated with occupation and environment, including accidents and violence; and differences associated with smoking and other behavioral risk factors.

Data are presented in Table 2.4 for life expectancy at birth and at age 65. Using age-65 data reduces the effects of risk factors at the younger ages, especially infant and childhood diseases. The mortality differential by sex exists even at age 65, suggesting a role for biological factors.

The United States falls fairly far down the list in life expectancy in the international comparison. In spite of spending substantially more dollars and a much greater percentage of GDP on health care, life expectancy remains significantly lower in the United States as compared to many other countries with advanced medical care systems. Even a number of industrialized countries that are less advanced than our own rank higher in longevity.

These international differentials are attributable largely to the greater degree of heterogeneity in our population, to various prominent risk factors in our society such as violence, and to economic barriers to obtaining health care services. In spite of spending substantially more of our economic pie on health care, however, the fact remains that our longevity is inferior to that of many other countries. It is especially important for the nation to focus on the needs of those subgroups in the population, such as the poor, who have high relative mortality.

Table 2.5 presents life expectancy data by race and sex for the United States since 1900. Data include life expectancy at birth and at age 65. Dramatic differentials have long been evident by sex and race. These differentials exist today owing

Table 2.4. Life Expectancy at Birth and at 65 Years of Age, According to Sex: Selected Countries 1998

Country	At Birth	At 65 Years
	Life expectancy in years (male)	
Australia	75.9	16.3
Bulgaria	67.4	12.5
Canada	76.0	16.3
Costa Rica	74.8	—
Cuba	75.8	—
England and Wales	75.1	15.5
France	74.8	16.4
Germany	74.5	15.3
Hong Kong	77.4	17.1
Israel	76.2	16.6
Japan	77.2	17.1
Puerto Rico	71.4	—
Russian Federation	61.4	11.6
Singapore	75.3	15.2
Spain	74.8	16.3
Sweden	76.9	16.3
Switzerland	76.3	16.6
United States	73.8	16.0
	Life expectancy in years (female)	
Australia	81.5	20.0
Bulgaria	74.7	15.1
Canada	81.5	20.1
Costa Rica	79.3	—
Cuba	78.2	—
England and Wales	80.0	18.7
France	82.4	20.9
Germany	80.6	19.0
Hong Kong	83.0	20.7
Israel	80.6	18.9
Japan	84.0	22.0
Puerto Rico	79.3	—
Russian Federation	73.3	15.5
Singapore	79.4	17.7
Spain	82.2	20.3
Sweden	81.9	20.0
Switzerland	82.4	20.5
United States	79.5	19.2

to biological, social, economic, genetic, and risk factors. Changes over time for all subgroups have also been dramatic, but for those aged 65 and older these changes have been much more moderate.

Mortality rates for the U.S. population, both current levels and projections for the future, are extremely important for policy purposes. For example, potential future costs of the Medicare and Medicaid programs, discussed in greater detail later in this book, are highly dependent on expectations of length of life. Without adjusting eligibility ages, the significantly increased expected length of life for U.S. males and females would result in tremendous additional costs for these programs. Recent increases in

ages for eligibility under the Social Security program were a direct phased-in response to these demographic trends. Recently, life expectancy tables used in the calculation of premiums for individual life insurance policies were adjusted to recognize the increase in life expectancies. Pricing of these policies is determined by, in large measure, risk of mortality in any given year for an individual based on sex and age. In this instance, increased longevity yields lower premium costs for the policies owing to lower year over year mortality risk.

Projections of mortality into the future carry considerable risk. Increasingly, biomedical knowledge is expanding such that more effective and significant interventions are feasible. This biomedical progress will yield increased length of life and may occur much sooner than originally expected. Threats of new disease, particularly infectious diseases, may endanger longevity for certain population groups. Increasing understanding of the genetic component of longevity may allow insurance companies to price policies with a component of genetic assessment built into premium determination. Such an action would also raise very complex social issues.

Table 2.5. Life Expectancy at Birth and at 65 Years of Age, According to Race and Sex: United States, Selected Years

Specified Age and Year	White		Black	
	Male	Female	Male	Female
At birth				
1900	46.6	48.7	32.5	33.5
1950	66.5	72.2	58.9	62.7
1960	67.4	74.1	60.7	65.9
1970	68.0	75.6	60.0	68.3
1980	70.7	78.1	63.8	72.5
1990	72.7	79.4	64.5	73.6
2000	74.8	80.0	68.2	74.9
At 65 years				
1900	11.5	12.2	10.4	11.4
1950	12.8	15.1	12.9	14.9
1960	12.9	15.9	12.7	15.1
1970	13.1	17.1	12.5	15.7
1980	14.2	18.4	13.0	16.8
1990	15.2	19.1	13.2	17.2
2000	16.3	19.2	14.5	17.4
At 75 years				
1980	8.8	11.5	8.3	10.7
1990	9.4	12.0	8.6	11.2
2000	10.1	12.1	9.4	11.2

Infant Mortality

A frequent measure of health status cited by policymakers and journalists is infant mortality. Unfortunately, infant mortality, defined as deaths in the first year of life, is actually a highly complex measure. Infant mortality is influenced by many factors, including, but certainly not limited to: access to prenatal medical care; biological factors attributable to both the mother and the fetus; factors associated with fetal development; genetics; social and environmental factors, including maternal nutrition; and likely many other factors which are not yet fully understood.

Differentials across countries in infant mortality, illustrated in Table 2.6, may result from many factors. The role of medical care in affecting infant mortality is itself an extremely complex issue.

Differences in health care systems across countries do not readily explain these differentials. In general, countries more advanced economically and socially and those with greater homogeneity in their population have lower infant mortality. With all the factors involved, it is difficult to conclude that differences in health care systems explain infant mortality differences between such countries as Japan and Sweden.

Of considerable interest are changes over time and differentials by age and race for infant mortality in the United States. These data are presented in Table 2.7.

Infant mortality has declined dramatically in the United States since 1950. In addition, significant differentials exist between various population groups, seen in the comparison of white and black infant mortality rates. These differentials are likely the result of the complex factors mentioned previ-

ously, such as less access to prenatal and obstetrical care and differences in economic status, nutrition, and lifestyles.

Reductions over time in infant mortality have been achieved in the United States through both societal economic advancements and medical care interventions. Improvements in standards of living and in education levels and better health habits have certainly contributed to enhanced

Table 2.6. Infant Mortality Rates and International Rankings: Selected Countries, Selected Years 1960–1999

Country	1960	1980	1999
	Infant deaths per 1,000 live births		
Australia	20.2	10.7	5.7
Canada	27.3	10.4	5.3
Cuba	37.3	19.6	6.4
England and Wales	22.5	12.1	5.8
France	27.5	10.0	4.3
Germany	35.0	12.4	4.5
Israel	31.0	15.2	5.7
Italy	43.9	14.6	5.1
Japan	30.7	7.5	3.4
Puerto Rico	43.3	18.5	10.6
Romania	75.7	29.3	18.6
Russian Federation	—	22.0	17.1
Singapore	34.8	11.7	3.5
Spain	43.7	12.3	4.5
Sweden	16.6	6.9	3.4
Switzerland	21.1	9.1	4.6
United States	26.0	12.6	7.1

Table 2.7. Infant Mortality Rates, According to Neonatal and Postneonatal Mortality Rates, by Race: United States, Selected Years

Race, Year	Total	Neonatal Under 28 Days	Neonatal Under 7 Days	Postneonatal 1 Month to 1 Year After Birth
	Deaths per 1,000 live births			
All races				
1950	29.2	20.5	17.8	8.7
1960	26.0	18.7	16.7	7.3
1970	20.0	15.1	13.6	4.9
1980	12.6	8.5	7.1	4.1
1990	9.2	5.8	4.8	3.4
2000	6.9	4.6	3.7	2.3
Race of child: white				
1950	26.8	19.4	17.1	7.4
1960	22.9	17.2	15.6	5.7
1970	17.8	13.8	12.5	4.0
1980	11.0	7.5	6.2	3.5
1990	7.7	4.9	4.0	2.8
2000	5.7	3.8	3.0	1.9
Race of child: black				
1950	43.9	27.8	23.0	16.1
1960	44.3	27.8	23.7	16.5
1970	32.6	22.8	20.3	9.9
1980	21.4	14.1	11.9	7.3
1990	17.0	10.9	9.2	6.1
2000	14.1	9.4	7.6	4.7

fetal outcomes. At the same time, direct medical care services have also clearly contributed to better maternal and fetal health. These medical care factors include better quality obstetrical and surgical services; enhanced monitoring technologies, particularly electronic fetal monitoring, which has increased the Caesarian section rate and improved fetal outcomes; less reliance on mechanically assisted deliveries; better drugs for the complications of pregnancy and delivery as well as for the postpartum period; and greatly enhanced ability to provide highly sophisticated care to premature infants using neonatal and intensive care units.

Technology is a two-edged sword, and the increased use of technology, particularly electronic fetal monitoring, has also contributed to a much higher percentage of deliveries being performed through Caesarian section rather than vaginal delivery. Over the past 30 years, the percentage of deliveries in the United States performed surgically using Caesarian section has increased from approximately 4.5 percent to approximately 25 percent. The increase in Caesarian sections is probably the result of technology and economics. Recently, there have been renewed efforts to focus the use of monitoring technologies on high-risk women.

Even more remarkable has been the reduction in maternal mortality in the United States even as recently as the period from 1970 to the present (Table 2.8). However, disturbing racial differentials still exist. And higher maternal age is not the risk factor that it once was.

Other factors, such as the availability of subspecialists in high-risk obstetrics and pediatrics practices, have contributed to this remarkable improvement in infant health. The relatively high rate of legal, therapeutic, induced abortions is also thought to have contributed to better neonatal and fetal outcomes owing to the disproportionate abortion rate among higher-risk, and particularly younger, women.

Approximately 1.3 million induced abortions are performed in the United States annually

Table 2.8. Maternal Mortality Rates for Complications of Pregnancy, Childbirth, and the Puerperium, by Race and Age: United States, Selected Years

Race and Age	1950	1970	1990	2000
	Number of deaths			
All persons	2,960	803	343	396
	Deaths per 100,000 live births			
White				
All ages, age adjusted	53.1	14.5	5.1	6.2
All ages, crude	61.1	14.4	5.4	7.5
Under 20 years	44.9	13.9	—	—
20–24 years	35.7	8.4	3.9	5.6
25–29 years	45.0	11.2	4.8	5.9
30–34 years	75.9	18.8	5.0	7.1
35 years and over	174.1	59.6	12.6	18.0
Black				
All ages, age adjusted	—	64.3	21.7	20.1
All ages, crude	—	59.8	22.4	22.0
Under 20 years	—	31.8	—	—
20–24 years	—	41.0	14.7	15.3
25–29 years	—	63.8	14.9	21.8
30–34 years	—	115.6	44.2	34.8
35 years and over	—	204.7	79.7	62.8

(Table 2.9) compared to almost four million live births. The number of induced abortions performed in the United States prior to the 1973 Supreme Court ruling, which facilitated access to abortion services nationally, is extremely difficult to estimate. And the exact role of induced abortion in affecting fetal mortality is also very difficult to estimate.

Although for the years indicated in Table 2.9 the most frequent method of surgical abortion is vacuum curettage, changes in technology are significantly impacting abortion practice in the United States and in other developed countries. Medically induced abortion and abortion performed much

Table 2.9. Legal Abortions, According to Selected Characteristics: United States, Selected Years

Characteristic	1973	1980	1990	1999
	Number reported (in thousands)			
	616	1,298	1,429	862
	Percentage distribution			
Period of gestation				
Under 9 weeks	36.1	51.7	51.6	57.6
9–10 weeks	29.4	26.2	25.3	20.2
11–12 weeks	17.9	12.2	11.7	10.2
13–15 weeks	6.9	5.2	6.4	6.2
16–20 weeks	8.0	3.9	4.0	4.3
21 weeks and over	1.7	0.9	1.0	1.5
Previous induced abortions				
0	67.6	58.1	57.1	53.7
1	23.5	26.5	26.9	27.1
2 or more	8.9	15.4	16.0	19.2

earlier in pregnancy are complicating the accuracy of data collection. Many of these abortions occur outside of a monitored surgical environment and the number of abortions may be difficult to determine. Political opposition to the relatively open access to abortion services that exists in the United States continues at various levels. Such opposition could potentially lead to more significant restrictions on the availability of these services in the future, particularly those accessed through surgical environments.

In addition to therapeutic induced abortion, whether by surgical or medical means, significant fetal loss also occurs as the result of spontaneous abortion. The frequency of spontaneous abortion is extremely difficult to estimate but a surprisingly high percentage of conceptions do result in spontaneous abortion as a result of biological processes. Spontaneous abortion may also lead to incomplete abortion or other consequences that require medical intervention. The analysis of fertility behavior is interesting, and important demographic, sociologi-

cal, and medical care perspectives on many components of such behavior have significant implications for the nature and future of our society. Differential fertility by population groups, for example, will to a large measure determine the future ethnic composition of the nation's population. Reproductive behaviors impact the health status of both men and women, disease patterns, and even the health of future generations.

CAUSES OF DEATH

Much can be learned from examining reported causes of death and illness for a population. Mortality, or death data, include number and cause of deaths by characteristic of the population. Morbidity refers to illness and disease, rather than death.

Tables 2.10 and 2.11 present death rates for the major causes of death for males and females and whites and blacks in the United States. Cancer, heart disease, and stroke are the three most common causes of death in the United States at the present time and have been for quite a number of years. The data are also presented for selected subgroups of the population.

These tables illustrate, for both males and females and whites and blacks, generally declining rates of mortality for the major causes of death. Particularly notable are reductions in mortality from cardiovascular disease, probably attributable in large measure to the introduction of new treatment modalities and certain preventive measures such as lifestyle changes, and drug treatments for hypertension and high cholesterol. Some other categories of disease, particularly cancers, have not experienced such notable reductions. In addition, many challenges remain as reflected in these data, such as the still high mortality rates in all categories and the great, unfortunate losses attributable to accident, suicide, homicide, and other nonphysiological causes. Newer challenges, such as the acquired immunodeficiency syndrome (AIDS) epidemic and increased mortality attributable to diabetes, are also evident. Generally

Table 2.10. Age-Adjusted Death Rates for Selected Causes of Death, According to Sex, Selected Years

Sex, Race, Hispanic Origin, and Cause of Death	1950	1980	2000
	\multicolumn{3}{c}{Age-adjusted death rate per 100,000 population}		
Male			
All causes	1,674.2	1,348.1	1,053.8
Diseases of heart	697.0	538.9	320.0 1
Ischemic heart disease	—	459.7	241.4 3
Cerebrovascular diseases	186.4	102.2	62.4 4
Malignant neoplasms	208.1	271.2	248.9 2
Trachea, bronchus, and lung	24.6	85.2	76.7 5
Colon, rectum, and anus	—	32.8	25.1
Prostate	28.6	32.8	30.4 8
Chronic lower respiratory diseases	—	49.9	55.8 6
Influenza and pneumonia	55.0	42.1	28.9 8
Chronic liver disease and cirrhosis	15.0	21.3	13.4
Diabetes mellitus	18.8	18.1	27.8
Human immunodeficiency virus (HIV) disease	—	—	7.9
Unintentional injuries	101.8	69.0	49.3 7
Motor vehicle-related injuries	38.5	33.6	21.7
Suicide	21.2	19.9	17.7
Homicide	7.9	16.6	9.0
Female			
All causes	1,236.0	817.9	731.4
Diseases of heart	484.7	320.8	210.9 1
Ischemic heart disease	—	263.1	146.5 3
Cerebrovascular diseases	175.8	91.7	59.1 4
Malignant neoplasms	182.3	166.7	167.6 2
Trachea, bronchus, and lung	5.8	24.4	41.3 5
Colon, rectum, and anus	—	23.8	17.7 10
Breast	31.9	31.9	26.8 7
Chronic lower respiratory diseases	—	14.9	37.4 6
Influenza and pneumonia	41.9	25.1	20.7
Chronic liver disease and cirrhosis	7.8	9.9	6.2
Diabetes mellitus	27.0	18.0	23.0 8
HIV disease	—	—	2.5
Unintentional injuries	54.0	26.1	22.0 9
Motor vehicle-related injuries	11.5	11.8	9.5
Suicide	5.6	5.7	4.0
Homicide	2.4	4.4	2.8

Table 2.11. Age-Adjusted Death Rates for Selected Causes of Death, According to Race, Selected Years

Sex, Race, Hispanic Origin, and Cause of Death	1950	1980	2000
	Age-adjusted death rate per 100,000 population		
White			
All causes	1,410.8	1,012.7	849.8
Diseases of heart	584.8	409.4	253.4
Ischemic heart disease	—	347.6	185.6
Cerebrovascular diseases	175.5	93.2	58.8
Malignant neoplasms	194.6	204.2	197.2
Trachea, bronchus, and lung	15.2	49.2	56.2
Colon, rectum, and anus	—	27.4	20.3
Prostate	28.4	30.5	27.8
Breast	32.4	32.1	26.3
Chronic lower respiratory diseases	—	29.3	46.0
Influenza and pneumonia	44.8	30.9	23.5
Chronic liver disease and cirrhosis	11.5	13.9	9.6
Diabetes mellitus	22.9	16.7	22.8
Human immunodeficiency virus (HIV) disease	—	—	2.8
Unintentional injuries	77.0	45.3	35.1
Motor vehicle-related injuries	24.4	22.6	15.6
Suicide	13.9	13.0	11.3
Homicide	2.6	6.7	3.6
Black or African American			
All causes	1,722.1	1,314.8	1,121.4
Diseases of heart	586.7	455.3	324.8
Ischemic heart disease	—	334.5	218.3
Cerebrovascular diseases	233.6	129.1	81.9
Malignant neoplasms	176.4	256.4	248.5
Trachea, bronchus, and lung	11.1	59.7	64.0
Colon, rectum, and anus	—	28.3	28.2
Prostate	30.9	61.1	68.1
Breast	25.3	31.7	34.5
Chronic lower respiratory diseases	—	19.2	31.6
Influenza and pneumonia	76.7	34.4	25.6
Chronic liver disease and cirrhosis	9.0	25.0	9.4
Diabetes mellitus	23.5	32.7	49.5
HIV disease	—	—	23.3
Unintentional injuries	79.9	57.6	37.7
Motor vehicle-related injuries	26.0	20.2	15.7
Suicide	4.5	6.5	5.5
Homicide	28.3	39.0	20.5

higher mortality from many causes for males as compared to females helps explain the greater longevity experienced by women in the U.S. population. Significantly higher mortality for blacks as compared to whites is evident in many, although not all, disease categories. Differences in a number of categories including AIDS and homicide are particularly notable. These differences reflect substantial patterns of behavior in the population leading to differentials in exposure. These data greatly facilitate our understanding of the underlying challenges that we face as a nation and in the health care system.

Mortality data for the early part of the twentieth century would list the major causes of death as including pneumonia, nephritis, and other infectious diseases, especially tuberculosis. This shift in deaths from infectious to chronic disease is probably the single most notable overall change in mortality patterns for the United States during the twentieth century.

Many infectious diseases have been controlled or eliminated entirely (Table 2.12). Vaccination and immunization and effective therapeutic interventions, particularly drugs, have enhanced our ability to combat infectious disease. The impact of the control of communicable and infectious diseases is dramatic, as reflected in this table. Diseases that once ravaged our population, particularly children, now represent a minimal risk. As more people live longer, chronic diseases have become more prevalent as causes of death.

It is important to recognize that infectious disease still causes significant mortality in the United States. This threat is dramatically illustrated by data on acquired immunodeficiency syndrome, or AIDS (Table 2.13). AIDS is a controllable, infectious disease for which we have only partial curative interventions at the present time.

Mortality associated with AIDS is significant, although AIDS is not one of the top five causes of death in the United States. AIDS is particularly prominent among young adults and those in various high–risk groups where it often is the leading cause of death.

AIDS mortality is decreasing as a result of new drug interventions, but the cost of these drugs is high and their long–term effectiveness is not yet known. The threat from the epidemic will persist in the future. AIDS is a preventable disease whose modes of transmission have been well elucidated and are primarily the result of lifestyles and behaviors. Preventive efforts and blood screening are clearly effective in reducing the virulence of the epidemic, although numerous social, behavioral, political, and economic factors complicate the picture.

Recent international experience with SARS (severe acute respiratory syndrome) dramatically jolted our complacency in facing the challenges of day-to-day life. This infectious disease caused governments in many developing and developed countries to take particular notice of the constant threats of new public health challenges. A relatively high mortality rate and ease of transmission suggests that our vigilance must be constant. The world-wide response to the SARS threat also dramatically illustrated the potential effectiveness of a rapid and coordinated international effort by public health officials to stop the spread of infectious disease. Many other challenges exist already such as the Ebola virus and other pathogenic organisms. Since September 11, 2001,

Table 2.12. Selected Notifiable Disease Cases: United States, Selected Years

Disease	1950	1970	2001
	Number of cases		
Diphtheria	5,796	435	2
Mumps	—	104,953	266
Pertussis (whooping cough)	120,718	4,249	7,580
Poliomyelitis	33,300	33	0
Rubella (German measles)	—	56,552	23
Rubeola (measles)	319,124	47,351	116
Tuberculosis	—	37,137	15,989
Syphilis	217,558	91,382	32,221
Gonorrhea	286,746	600,072	361,705

Table 2.13. Death Rates for Human Immunodeficiency Virus (HIV) Infection; According to Sex: United States, Selected Years

Sex	1987	1990	2000
	Deaths per 100,000 resident population		
Male			
All ages, age adjusted	10.0	17.7	7.9
All ages, crude	10.2	18.5	7.9
Under 1 year	2.2	2.4	—
1–4 years	0.7	0.8	—
5–14 years	0.2	0.3	0.1
15–24 years	2.2	2.2	0.5
25–34 years	20.7	34.5	8.0
35–44 years	26.3	50.2	19.8
45–54 years	15.5	29.1	17.8
55–64 years	6.8	12.0	8.7
65–74 years	2.4	3.7	3.8
75–84 years	1.2	1.1	1.3
85 years and over	—	—	—
Female			
All ages, age adjusted	1.1	2.1	2.5
All ages, crude	1.1	2.2	2.5
Under 1 year	2.5	3.0	—
1–4 years	0.7	0.8	—
5–14 years	—	0.2	0.1
15–24 years	0.3	0.7	0.4
25–34 years	2.8	4.9	4.2
35–44 years	2.1	5.2	6.5
45–54 years	0.8	1.9	4.4
55–64 years	0.5	1.1	1.8
65–74 years	0.5	0.8	0.8
75–84 years	0.5	0.4	0.3
85 years and over	—	—	—

the potential threat of terrorist activity involving biological or chemical agents is another ongoing reality that we face in our day-to-day lives against which our public health defenses must be vigilant at all times.

The challenges we face from nature and man-made threats in our world today will require a constant monitoring and readiness to respond henceforth.

In the United States, cardiovascular mortality has declined significantly over the past 30 years, as a result of more effective interventions, including coronary artery bypass surgery and better diagnosis. Prevention, drug interventions, healthier lifestyles, and better diets have had a role. Exercise has been shown to be important in reducing cardiovascular mortality. Overall, our ability to intervene using a variety of approaches in recent years has been greatly enhanced in the area of cardiovascular health.

Somewhat remarkably, survival experience from many forms of cancer has not improved significantly over the past 30 years. In general, with the exception of childhood leukemias and a number of other types of neoplastic disease, mortality rates have remained fairly high. This is in spite of better and earlier detection, more effective interventions for some types of malignant disease, and heightened public awareness. Improvement in nutrition and better scientific understanding and public awareness of dietary contributions to cancer prevention probably have had only a minor impact on cancer incidence and mortality. Environmental and occupational exposures have certainly contributed to some forms of neoplastic disease, but the total contribution from environmental factors is most certainly less than generally perceived.

Health behaviors, and particularly cigarette and tobacco product consumption, discussed further below, are extremely important contributors to the incidence of, and mortality associated with, many cancers, cardiovascular diseases, and other illnesses. Cancer mortality patterns, although perhaps perplexing, reflect the aging of the population and greater susceptibility to the long-term effects of carcinogenic factors, and the lack, until recently, of a fundamental biological understanding of neoplastic disease processes that could lead to more successful interventions.

Table 2.14 presents 5-year survival data for selected cancer sites compiled from recent data.

The data are derived from selected regional cancer registries since no national data are available.

Table 2.14. Five-Year Relative Cancer Survival Rates for Selected Sites, According to Race and Sex: Selected Geographic Areas, Selected Years

Sex and Site	White		Black	
	1974–79	1992–98	1974–79	1992–98
Male				
All sites	43.4	63.5	32.1	54.0
Oral cavity and pharynx	54.4	57.8	31.2	29.5
Esophagus	5.2	14.7	2.3	9.0
Stomach	13.8	19.5	15.3	19.2
Colon	51.0	63.0	45.4	53.2
Rectum	48.9	61.6	36.7	51.6
Pancreas	2.6	4.3	2.4	4.2
Lung and bronchus	11.6	13.3	10.0	10.8
Prostate gland	70.3	97.8	60.8	92.6
Urinary bladder	75.9	84.4	58.9	69.4
Non-Hodgkin's lymphoma	47.2	52.7	44.7	41.4
Leukemia	35.6	48.4	30.7	37.9
Female				
All sites	57.4	64.2	46.9	51.0
Colon	52.6	62.4	48.7	52.5
Rectum	50.7	63.5	43.8	53.8
Pancreas	2.3	4.4	4.1	3.7
Lung and bronchus	16.7	17.0	15.5	14.7
Melanoma of skin	85.8	91.8	69.9	61.9
Breast	75.4	87.6	63.1	72.5
Cervix uteri	69.7	72.1	63.0	59.9
Corpus uteri	87.7	86.0	59.4	60.5
Ovary	37.2	52.5	40.5	52.5
Non-Hodgkin's lymphoma	49.3	60.2	57.5	53.8

Slowly, progress in the battle against various forms of cancer is being achieved. The complexity of the challenge is immense but clinical research is beginning to yield drug interventions that are at least moderately effective against certain types of cancer. Cancer is a generic disease category that covers many, many types of illnesses, and the immense biological complexity of processes involved in the development of various types of cancer represents a great challenge to our biomedical research community.

In addition to some successes in the primarily pharmaceutical approach to treating certain types of cancer, increasing progress is also being achieved in the area of prevention. Prevention of both primary cancer occurrence and recidivism for patients who have already successfully battled cancer is a high priority in our national effort to moderate the impact of this devastating disease category. Primary prevention has particularly benefited in recent years from a much greater understanding of the epidemiological basis of cancer occurrence, including both patterns of cancer incidence in communities and associated genetic, environmental, and other risk factors, as well as a better understanding of the behavioral and biological factors associated with increased risk of cancer for any one individual.

Cancer progress illustrates dramatically the benefits of expenditures over the past 30 years on basic research focusing on molecular biology. Prior to such directed effort at understanding the underlying biology of disease, cancer intervention consisted more of screening, detection, and surgical removal with relatively little targeted treatment that recognized the actual physiological processes involved in the disease. Now we are embarking on a new era of cancer detection, screening, prevention, and treatment that is much more attuned to the underlying biological processes involved and that ultimately, with time, will be much more effective in preventing, treating, and eliminating this threat from our daily life.

A Note on Race and Other Differentials

From a public health and health services perspective it is particularly important to emphasize differentials in morbidity, mortality, and other measures of illness and disease based on race and other social demographic and economic variables. Throughout this chapter selected racial differentials have been noted. In the real world, such differences by various population groups are quite common across many of the health status and health care indicators illustrated in this chapter. The development of targeted programs in health care delivery, public health, and health promotion to specific population groups whose health indicators suggest deficiencies in access to health care or understanding of health behaviors is particularly important. Numerous examples of the importance of examining populations by their characteristics in developing targeted interventions exist. For example, as indicated in this chapter, violence and accidents are much more common among blacks and certain other minority groups and among young men than for other population groups, suggesting opportunities for targeted public health interventions. Hypertension and certain other diseases may be more common among various population subgroups such that education and medical interventions targeting these populations with information regarding diet, exercise, and possible preventive use of pharmacological agents are warranted. As discussed further later, the recent public health emphasis on controlling the epidemic of obesity and the traditional public health focus on smoking are further illustrations of population needs for which targeted efforts can be directed toward those groups in the population at highest risk of developing disease based on their personal behaviors and lifestyles. For example, alcohol use among American Indians increases the risk of accidents and a variety of illnesses and targeted interventions can be highly beneficial in reducing morbidity and mortality.

Healthy Behaviors and Lifestyles

Many other patterns of behavior and lifestyle also contribute to population mortality and morbidity. More than 40,000 people are killed and approximately 2 million people are injured annually in vehicular accidents in the United States. Table 2.15 presents data on motor vehicle accidents in the United States by age and sex. Although vehicular mortality has declined substantially per 100,000 resident population, the numbers are still shocking. Rates and numbers of deaths are particularly high for the young adult and older population groups and for males. Since we have considerable knowledge about how to build safer cars, safer highways, and how to educate and enforce safer driving, there is no excuse for such carnage on the highway.

Approximately one third to one half of all vehicular fatalities are associated with drug and alcohol consumption. Effective, although inconvenient, enforcement methods could significantly reduce these tragic losses. Compromises in individual freedom are needed if we want to provide greater safety and security on the nation's roads. Most people would agree that this mayhem is unacceptable in a technologically advanced society. Thus far, however, we have lacked the will, and our politicians have lacked the courage, to stop it.

Another unfortunate cause of mortality in the United States is homicide. Table 2.16 presents data related to this cause of death. For most population groups reflected in this table, mortality associated with homicide has increased substantially over the past half century. Comparing the data for younger, white males with those for younger, black males, the mortality rate associated with homicide for this latter group is especially alarming. For black males ages 15 to 44, mortality associated with homicide is approximately five to seven times greater than that for the comparable population of white males. This reflects a truly tragic situation for the nation and one that must be addressed by broad social and economic interventions.

Table 2.15. Death Rates for Motor Vehicle-Related Injuries, According to Sex and Age: United States, Selected Years

Sex and Age	1950	2000
	Deaths per 100,000 resident population	
Male		
All ages, age adjusted	38.5	21.7
Under 1 year	9.1	4.6
1–14 years	12.3	4.9
1–4 years	13.0	4.7
5–14 years	11.9	5.0
15–24 years	56.7	37.4
15–19 years	46.3	33.9
20–24 years	66.7	41.2
25–34 years	40.8	25.5
35–44 years	32.5	22.0
45–64 years	37.7	20.2
45–54 years	33.6	20.4
55–64 years	43.1	19.8
65 years and older	66.6	29.5
64–74 years	59.1	21.7
75–84 years	85.0	35.6
85 years and older	78.1	57.5
Female		
All ages, age adjusted	11.5	9.5
Under 1 year	7.6	4.2
1–14 years	7.2	3.7
1–4 years	10.0	3.8
5–14 years	5.7	3.6
15–24 years	12.6	15.9
15–19 years	12.9	17.5
20–24 years	12.2	14.2
25–34 years	9.3	8.8
35–44 years	8.5	8.8
45–64 years	12.6	8.7
45–54 years	10.9	8.2
55–64 years	14.9	9.5
65 years and older	21.9	15.8
64–74 years	20.6	12.3
75–84 years	25.2	19.2
85 years and older	22.1	19.3

It has been estimated that approximately 450,000 deaths a year in the United States are caused by the consumption of tobacco products. The long-term effects of tobacco consumption on a society's mortality experience is a very complicated issue. Nevertheless, it is certain that these products have significantly and adversely impacted the health of the population in this country and throughout the world.

Table 2.17 illustrates the dramatic decline in cigarette smoking in the United States since 1965. Although epidemiological evidence implicating tobacco products in various forms of cancer, coronary artery disease, and other illnesses has existed since the 1940s, the report of the Surgeon General of the United States in 1964 marked a turning point in official governmental policy and in public recognition of the risks inherent in the use of these products.

Over the past 30 years, public awareness of these risks has led to a decline in tobacco consumption and restrictions on the marketing of tobacco products. Recent evidence concerning the adverse consequences of secondhand tobacco exposure has heightened opposition to tobacco products. International consumption, on the other hand, has continued to expand, with an emphasis on the higher-risk forms of the product, such as unfiltered, high-tar, and high-nicotine cigarettes.

Cigarette consumption has declined as a result of heightened public awareness of health risks, increasing taxation, and regulation, particularly of advertising. Tobacco products dramatically illustrate the public policy challenges involved in trading off personal freedom against societal needs. Consumption of tobacco products clearly leads to adverse health consequences and limitations on life spans. Our society has established barriers to tobacco consumption, such as age restrictions for the purchase of products. However, we have not made these products illegal to produce or consume. Public education, combined with limited market interventions, is currently the strategy of choice in containing the adverse consequences of these products.

Recent legal assaults on the tobacco industry have resulted in huge settlement payments to government.

These settlements have also resulted in higher product prices. The battle against this industry will continue for years in the courts and in the media.

Excessive alcohol consumption, which also has significant adverse health consequences and huge costs for our society, also illustrates the trade-off of individual freedom against the public welfare. These trade-offs are increasingly important as government's role in paying the nation's health care bill expands, and with our expectations for enhanced longevity and a healthier environment in which to live.

During Prohibition, government tried to stop the production of alcohol products. The political

Table 2.16. Death Rates for Homicide, According to Sex, Race, and Age: United States, Selected Years

Sex, Race, and Age	1950	1980	2001
	Deaths per 100,000 resident population		
White males			
All ages, age adjusted	3.8	10.4	7.1
Under 1 year	4.3	4.3	7.3
1–14 years	0.4	1.2	1.1
15–24 years	3.2	15.1	11.2
25–44 years	5.4	17.2	11.5
25–34 years	4.9	18.5	12.3
35–44 years	6.1	15.2	10.7
45–64 years	4.8	9.8	6.4
65 years and older	3.8	6.7	3.0
Black males			
All ages, age adjusted	47.0	69.4	36.2
Under 1 year	—	18.6	21.0
1–14 years	1.8	4.1	3.6
15–24 years	53.8	82.6	85.7
25–44 years	92.8	130.0	58.1
25–34 years	104.3	142.9	78.8
35–44 years	80.0	109.3	38.5
45–64 years	46.0	70.6	22.7
65 years and older	16.5	30.9	11.5

Table 2.17. Current Cigarette Smoking by Persons 18 Years of Age and Older, According to Sex and Age: United States, Selected Years

Sex and Age	1965	1985	2001
	Percentage of persons who are current cigarette smokers		
18 years and older, age adjusted			
All persons	41.9	29.9	22.7
Male	51.2	32.2	24.7
Female	33.7	27.9	20.8
White male	50.4	31.3	24.9
Black or African American male	58.8	40.2	27.6
White female	33.9	27.9	22.1
Black or African American female	31.8	30.9	17.9

and economic failures of this policy raises questions about government regulation of lifestyles. Current strategies to deal with violence, illicit drug use, auto safety, and sexual behavior illustrate other visible failures of governmental intervention in people's lives to promote their health.

We must decide how far we want government to go in protecting us from ourselves. We must determine which specific mechanisms will be used to achieve health promotion objectives. These are difficult issues for the nation's politicians to address; they fear alienating voters. However, since so much morbidity and mortality are attributable to lifestyle, behavior, nutrition, and environment, containing costs and promoting health mandate that we face these issues head on.

The relationships between health and the social and economic aspects of our society are so strong that improving the mental and physical health of our population requires that we address broader societal ills. Approximately one million children are born annually to unmarried women; the divorce rate is approximately half of the marriage rate; about one fourth of all Americans live alone; a minority of children live in a traditional family with their biological parents; poverty and malnutrition are rampant; and social decay, violence, and stress permeate our society.

We do more talking than acting in promoting healthy lifestyles and behaviors; our consumption of fat, cholesterol, and salt in our diets is still far too great; and many other aspects of our economic, social, and psychological well-being remain deficient. The environment and the workplace both leave much to be desired in promoting our physiological and psychological well-being. Even our spiritual health is being constantly challenged.

Yet, for all that is wrong in our society, we are still a nation full of hope and enthusiasm, of incredible strength and financial resources, of creativity and accomplishment. We must harness our great resources and our many strengths in the pursuit of health and happiness in order to recognize and work toward a vision of a healthier, happier nation.

Each individual in our society must assume greater personal responsibility for his or her own health. Our national energies must be directed toward creating a world dedicated to the pursuit of a better life for all Americans.

THE ULTIMATE RESPONSIBILITY: HEALTHY LIFESTYLES

Although the empirical evidence is still limited in relating aspects of lifestyles to health, we are increasingly able to identify attributes of living that are associated with greater longevity. One well-known epidemiologist identified seven characteristics of individuals who tend to live longer. Such individuals do not smoke; get enough sleep; eat breakfast; avoid excessive weight; use alcohol in moderation or not at all; exercise; and do not eat (bad) snacks!

The evidence is certainly accumulating in support of: avoiding stress; exercising; avoiding excessive weight; consuming a proper diet; limiting consumption of alcohol; eliminating consumption of tobacco products; avoiding risky behaviors, particularly those involving sexual activity, drug and alcohol consumption, including abuse of legal and illegal drugs; reducing exposure to violence; and maintaining good driving habits. Perhaps 15 to 20 percent of all mortality in the country is attributable to behavior. Even such tried and tested contributors to health as immunization and vaccination show astoundingly poor compliance in communities throughout the country.

We cannot rely on government to do its part in protecting health if we as individuals fail to do our parts. We cannot expect to be rescued from every source of morbidity and mortality by the nation's health care system if we do not individually and collectively emphasize prevention of disease and illness in the first place. That is part of the challenge that we face as professionals and as responsible citizens.

STUDY QUESTIONS

1. What has been the pattern of population growth in the United States over the past 200 years?
2. How did fertility rates change in the United States during the twentieth century?
3. Why do women live longer than men?
4. Why do Americans have a shorter average life span than people in many other countries of the world?
5. What were the patterns of infant mortality in the United States and, by comparison, in other countries of the world during the twentieth century?
6. What are the major causes of death in the United States at the present time, focusing on the top ten causes for males and for females?
7. For which causes of death is mortality higher among blacks than whites, and what are the reasons for these differences?
8. How does mortality from AIDS compare to other causes of death in the United States?
9. How did preventable causes of death, such as alcohol consumption, cigarette consumption, and vehicular accidents contribute to the nation's patterns of mortality in the twentieth century?

CHAPTER 3

Access to Health Care Services

Chapter Objectives

1. To interpret the role of access.
2. To assess access to health care.
3. To explore measures of access.

The concept of access to health care services is of vital importance. Measuring, interpreting, and assessing a population's access to health care services is a key component of policy analysis. Such analysis can help determine the successes or failures of a health care system, and can be used to assess additional system needs.

Indeed, access to health care has been one of the fundamental themes in the social and political environment of the United States for the last 100 years. Concerns over financial access to care have led to a fundamental change in the role of government with the passage of the Medicare program legislation and to a lesser extent, the Medicaid program. Ensuring access to care for those in the greatest need of services has always been a fundamental concern of government but this mandate has expanded substantially since the 1960s. The government's role in assessing and improving access to care has also extended to many other components of the health care system such as emergency services, preventive and public health measures, and targeted services for specific populations such as youth and children as well as pregnant women. Most recently, access concerns have revolved around Medicare outpatient drug coverage, the uninsured, reductions in benefits and coverage for the insured, and availability of all types of resources for all citizens. Access issues will, in one form or another, always be on the front burner of policy analysis and decision makers in health care.

FACTORS ASSOCIATED WITH ACCESS TO HEALTH CARE

Numerous factors affect access to health care services. These include environmental issues such as the forces at work in a society that are associated with health service needs. Environment includes, but is certainly not limited to, accidents and violence, lifestyles, general economic well-being, levels of stress, and societal perspectives on the role and use of health services.

The nature and structure of the health care system are also significant factors in affecting access to health services. Most recently, the restructuring of the health care system based on the principles of managed care has substantially changed access to services, often intentionally. The system's structure, and the organization and financing of the components of the system, are major determinants of access to health care and are key themes throughout this book.

A variety of population characteristics and individual attributes impacts access to health services. These include economic factors such as financial wealth and levels of insurance coverage. Also relevant is the availability of health services in an individual's community, as measured by such factors as physician-to-population and hospital bed-to-population ratios. Individuals' preexisting conditions and health status, of course, are also extremely important contributors to the need for care and to access. These factors are often measured in conjunction with demographic variables such as age and sex.

In our increasingly heterogeneous society, access is also affected by an ever-expanding array of issues and situations. These include communication needs of populations who do not speak or whose primary language is not English. Even individuals who speak some English may not be able to describe signs and symptoms accurately to health care providers in English or may not be understood adequately in their native tongue. Cultural attitudes and assimilation issues also impact interaction with the nation's health care system on the part of many individuals, sometimes even leading to a lack of trust in the provider network.

Impressions regarding health care and attitudes toward physical and mental signs and symptoms are important determinants of access. For example, it has long been demonstrated that different population subgroups react differently to various symptoms, such as pain, in deciding whether to seek health care. Social structure, education, occupation, and ethnicity are all associated with how people respond to their own health concerns, and to the health care system itself. Some individuals are more likely to respond to serious signs and symptoms than are others. Some people perceive the health care system to be more responsive to their needs, and thus seek care more readily than do other individuals. These factors are compounded by such issues as social structure and interpersonal networks and contacts. Studies of physicians' spouses illustrate, for example, that these individuals are often more likely to seek care because of their closer ties to the health care system.

Health care beliefs involving attitudes, values, and knowledge for individuals are aggregated into more generalizable community-based summaries. As a result, behavior can vary between communities based on the composition of their populations. Thus, no one template for providing health care services is likely to be equally applicable to all communities in our nation. Rather, the structure of health care services must be tailored to the needs of each community and its citizens. The highly complex and heterogeneous nature of our society guarantees that ensuring health care for all Americans will always be difficult. Additional complexity arises from human behavior such as assuring that patients comply with medical regimens and follow their physicians' orders as to diet, nutrition, and other lifestyle contributors to health.

DIFFERENT TYPES OF ACCESS TO HEALTH CARE

Numerous measures of access to health care are utilized in assessing the successes or failures of the nation's health care system. The most easily understood of these is realized access, which measures actual utilization of health care services. Measures of realized access include, for example, the number of physician visits per person or per population, hospital bed days utilized, and other indicators of actual utilization.

As noted elsewhere, access is achieved. Need and demand factors are mitigated by financial and other barriers to obtaining care. Assessing the extent to which access is inhibited, for whom, and under what conditions is a key aspect of analysis conducted by policymakers seeking to improve the system. For example, impressions that financial factors such as lack of health insurance or income are deficient for various population groups led to such major programs as Medicare and Medicaid. Determining that physical access is limited by geographic considerations might lead to the construction of additional physical facilities, or the dispersion of resources more broadly within a community. Hours of operation might be modified or triaging might be improved to increase access to care as well.

Access problems can lead to poorer health status, delays in obtaining care, and episodic or fragmented services. Lack of continuity, duplication of services, and wastefulness of resources are other complications of access deficiencies. Improving personal practices and attitudes is an important component of dealing with access issues. Health promotion and education provide patients with information about illness and disease, improve compliance with medical regimens and treatments, and, of course, ultimately encourage healthy lifestyles involving diet, exercise, and stress management.

Access issues also involve the efficient use of health care resources. It is important not only to ensure access, but also to control access in such a way that resources are rationally allocated and carefully utilized in the provision of care. This is the area in which managed care organizations have striven, thus far not completely successfully, to improve the operation of the health care system. Future improvements in the organization of the health care system must ensure that we utilize national resources as efficiently as possible, while at the same time striving to improve the quality of care for patients in the system.

MEASURES OF ACCESS TO HEALTH CARE

Table 3.1 illustrates how access to health care services can be measured for a population. Although not totally inclusive, the measures in this table illustrate the broad scope of indicators utilized to assess access in a population. Comparison of these measures across different geographic regions or population segments is utilized to indicate barriers that may require further intervention, such as the construction of additional facilities or the expansion of entitlement programs.

Ronald Andersen pioneered the analytical approaches to conceptualizing and analyzing access to health care services. He outlined a structure for visualizing access that considered such factors as enabling variables that facilitated access to care and background variables such as social demographic status as well as health care attitudes and beliefs. Over the years, many others from a variety of disciplines have conceptualized and measured access to health care using a variety of approaches. However, from a practical perspective on a daily basis, measuring access typically focuses on more readily available variables such as social demographic characteristics of patients and measures of actual utilization of services. In recent years, more sophisticated approaches have also utilized newer technologies such as Geographic Information Systems (GIS), which, using computers, map physical access to the layout of cities, including freeways and other transportation routes. These more sophisticated approaches can also be valuable in determining the location of satellite clinics of hospitals and of emergency resources such as ambulance stations. Finally, an added area of analysis in measuring access has been to understand better the needs of the underinsured and uninsured in our population. These analyses focus on insurance coverage, financial resources, and other aspects of access as measured by financial indicators. The analysis of access to health care is a complex and multidisciplined endeavor that is continually evolving.

The analysis of access to health care is particularly important for specific services. Such indicators as the percentage of women obtaining breast cancer screening are utilized by national assessment organizations to assess the quality of care provided in managed care plans. Use of access measures such as these, which relate to specific services thought to be warranted for a particular population segment, can be especially useful in conducting evaluations of the quality of care provided. Of course, assessments must extend beyond purely whether care is provided or whether or not to include a determination of the quality and appropriateness of that care.

Table 3.1. Illustrative Measures of Access to Health Care

Access Area	Typical Access Measures
Health system	Physician-to-population ratio
	Hospital bed-to-population ratio
Financial	Per capita health care expenditures
	Percentage insurance coverage
Location	Physician office use measures
	Hospital use measures
Level	Ambulatory care use measures
	Inpatient hospital services use measures
	Long-term care/nursing home services use measures
Sociodemographic	Race and ethnicity differentials
	Education differentials
	Marital status differentials

ACCESS TRENDS OVER TIME

Time-based analysis of access trends is essential to track the evolution of the health care system. Measuring differential access by geographic areas or population subgroups effectively tells the policy analyst how changes in the health care system and in individuals' use of that system are translated into actual health care products. Table 3.2 illustrates some of the time-based access trends that are tracked to assess the health care system's development and efficiencies.

Table 3.2 illustrates the increased access to health care that has occurred since the introduction of national entitlement programs, including Medicare and Medicaid, in the 1960s. Those most affected include lower-income individuals whose utilization of health care, and, hence, access, as measured by hospital admissions and physician visits, has increased substantially. In recent years relative differentials across many population groups have moderated. Similarly, differences in indicators of access by race also show substantial change since the implementation of Medicare and Medicaid in the 1960s.

Extensive data are available from various surveys, especially those conducted by the federal government, for tracking changes in access to care for various population groups. This information is extremely valuable for national policymaking and contributes to the overall debate about the future of the health care system. Examples of current access-related issues reflected in these data include a lack of access to dental care for individuals without financial resources, a considerable percentage of the population that currently has no insurance coverage or is underinsured, and a lack of adequate access for many to long-term care and mental health services.

ACCESS ISSUES FOR THE FUTURE

Access is a key issue that has challenged our nation's health care system from its beginning. As a nation, we have long struggled with issues of who has the right to access health services, which services, and under what conditions. Assuring adequate access for care is an issue that permeates all aspects of health policy and delivery. Managed care organizations constantly struggle with the trade-offs involved in controlling access to care versus assuming increased costs. Social programs exist to address issues of access. Medicare and Medicaid have their origins in the realization that access to health care for some population groups had not met national social goals.

Conceptually, understanding differential access to care for various population groups, for different types of services, and in various settings in which care is provided is important for analyzing the nature and operation of the health care system. The formulation and measurement of indicators of access to care are challenging areas for health services researchers, but ones that contribute to improving the health care system. Addressing the challenges of access provides a key focal point for analyzing our goals as a nation.

Table 3.2. Illustrative Measures of Changes in Access to Care: United States, Selected Years

Measure	Year	
	Previous	Recent
Pap smear, women age 18 and older (percentage with test past 3 years)	74.1 (1987)	81.4 (2000)
Mammograms, women age 65 years and older (percentage are with test past 2 years)	22.8 (1987)	68.0 (2000)
Mammograms, black women age 40 years and older (percentage with test past 2 years)	24.0 (1987)	67.8 (2000)
Dental visits, Americans age 65 years and older (percentage with visit past year)	39.3 (1983)	56.3 (2001)

Issues of access are fundamental to the current discussions about reforming the nation's health care system. For example, the debate regarding coverage of pharmaceutical products under the Medicare program for outpatient services is fundamentally one about improving financial access to care. Discussion and a national advisory panel report on issues related to mental health services in the United States likewise focus on issues of access and concerns over fragmentation of the system entry points to seeking care and other access related issues.

Many of our concerns about health care relate in one manner or another to issues of access. The development of new technologies, therapies, and interventions ultimately translates into issues about who, what, when, and how people should have access to those benefits of our national biomedical efforts. Rationing services, drawing the line as to which services should be available to which population groups and under what circumstances, is ultimately an issue of access. Access is also intertwined with concerns regarding the costs of services and the ultimate political decisions that must be made regarding allocation of resources to population groups for purposes of receiving health care services.

Ultimately, it is the issues of access and cost that we must successfully address to ensure that all citizens receive a level of health care services that meets their most fundamental needs. It is also important to recognize that issues of access are intimately connected to factors associated with the quality of care; with satisfaction on the part of providers and consumers; and with national political, economic, and social goals.

STUDY QUESTIONS

1. What is access to health care?
2. How is access to health care measured?
3. What is the policy value of measuring access to health care?
4. What are five specific measures of utilization relevant to access to health care?
5. How is access an important issue in managed care?

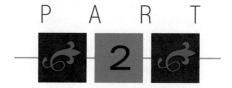

P A R T

2

Organizational and Individual Providers

This section describes the major settings in which health care services are provided. These include public health services, ambulatory care, institutional hospital services, long-term care, and mental health services.

CHAPTER 4

Ambulatory Health Services: Backbone of the System*

Chapter Objectives

1. To describe the scope and role of ambulatory care services in the United States.
2. To describe the types of services provided in ambulatory care settings.
3. To depict the role of preventive health services.
4. To outline the nature of group practice in the United States.
5. To examine the nature of physician-based office practice in the United States.
6. To explore new and innovative avenues for providing ambulatory care services.
7. To outline the organizational role and control mechanisms of ambulatory care services.
8. To assess the allocation of responsibility for coordination, integration, appropriateness, and rationalization between ambulatory care and other sectors.

*Reprinted and adapted from Introduction to Health Services, 6th Edition, edited by S. J. Williams and P. R. Torrens, 2002, Clifton Park, NY: Thomson Delmar Learning.

The evolution of our nation's health care system, particularly technological innovations in medicine and surgery, together with changes in financial arrangements, have shifted the focus of the provision and control of health services to the ambulatory care arena. For many years, the hospital was the principal focus of the health care delivery system. Over the past decade, the role of the hospital in controlling the delivery of health care has eroded while the advantages of shifting control and services to the ambulatory sector have been increasingly recognized by payers and providers alike. The ambulatory arena is likewise more tolerable for the patient as well.

This chapter addresses the historical development and current and future roles of ambulatory care services. It places these services in a broader context that recognizes both the direct provision of care and mechanisms of controlling patients and providers within various payment arrangements. Descriptions of various ambulatory care provider settings, quantitative descriptions of the volume and nature of such services, and the increasingly important role of these services in the coordination and organization of the system are addressed.

The role of ambulatory care services in organizing and rationalizing the health care system has been greatly enhanced by the rapid growth of managed care, by the changing nature and role of hospitals and hospital systems, and by enhancement of the gatekeeper and coordinating function of frontline providers of care. The increasing shift of many services that traditionally have been performed on an inpatient basis such as many surgical services, maintenance-oriented care that is now provided in the home rather than in the hospital, and other practical and technological changes have also heightened interest in ambulatory care. Finally, the increasing consolidation and vertical integration of the health care system is greatly increasing the linkages between ambulatory care and other services.

Tremendous operational and monetary pressures have been placed on ambulatory care services over the past few years as a result of managed care and other trends in the health care system. The past financial difficulties of physician-management companies and of other ambulatory care organizations highlight these pressures. Managers of these resources face an increasingly difficult environment. Physician and consumer dissatisfaction with many aspects of managed care, particularly those associated with control of physician practice patterns and behavior, has recently reached a crescendo. Technological advances that increasingly point toward the delivery of services through ambulatory care mechanisms will require organizational responses appropriate to the expanding role of this modality in the provision of care throughout the country.

Traditionally ambulatory care services have been viewed as the primary source of contact that most people have with the health care system. Although there are few concise definitions of ambulatory care, these services can be described as care provided to noninstitutionalized patients. Sometimes ambulatory care is termed care for the "walking patient." Ambulatory care includes a wide range of services, from simple, routine treatment to surprisingly complex tests and therapies.

HISTORICAL PERSPECTIVE AND TYPES OF CARE

Ambulatory care originated with the healing arts themselves. In primitive societies and for many years thereafter, until the advent of institutional care, all care was provided on what might be referred to as an *ambulatory care basis*. Of course, the types of care given then bear little resemblance to today's health care, but the history of civilization demonstrates a consistent commitment to caring for the sick, using whatever knowledge was available at the time. Remarkable forms of medical practice occurred in Greece, Rome, and other relatively sophisticated societies. In fact, many primitive societies had, and most, if not all, countries still have, their own indigenous practitioners such as religious healers and medicine men.

In more recent times, ambulatory care was provided in many new settings by a variety of more advanced practitioners. In Europe, and later in the United States, many of these services were made available to wealthy patients in their homes, while poor people were cared for in dispensaries and public clinics. With improvements in hospital care, more patients of all social classes received both inpatient and outpatient care in hospital settings. In the United States, the poor have always been more likely than wealthier people to obtain care from the hospital than from private physicians.

In the United States, ambulatory care services were traditionally provided by individual medical practitioners working in their offices and in patients' homes and by public clinics operating primarily for the benefit of poor and indigent patients. The limited technological equipment that physicians required allowed them to travel easily, carrying their principal supplies with them. Thus home care was common, especially among wealthier patients. Physicians' offices were frequently located in their homes or in other small buildings, as opposed to today's medical office buildings or large medical centers. The general practitioner who made house calls, provided guidance, and offered available treatments was typical of the state of primary care before World War II.

Since World War II, however, an explosion of medical knowledge has led to increasing specialization, more complex technology, and rapid changes in the setting and nature of services. Fewer physicians are able or willing to travel to the patient's home, and many can no longer carry with them the equipment and supplies or bring the specialized personnel available in an office. The growth of technical specialization, in particular, has led to the rapid expansion of new settings for providing care, such as group practices and, more recently, a profusion of specialized facilities. Increased knowledge has also led to the partial phasing out of the "traditional" general practitioner, although a new form of generalist is now

taking hold, encouraged by managed care and concerns over comprehensiveness of care.

For the poor, in both Europe and the United States, care, when available, was often limited to public or philanthropic clinics or dispensaries. Private practitioners may have given some of their time to serve the poor, but their devotion to the patient was probably limited, as was the availability of care and the facilities in which services were provided.

Early efforts to link ambulatory care services and integrate them formally with inpatient care were promoted in this country and in Europe, in part through the concept of regionalization. In Great Britain, the concept was presented in the Dawson Report, which eventually led to the formation of the National Health Service. In the United States, however, centralization of the health care system under federal authority has not been accepted as a politically viable alternative, as evident in the rejection of the Clinton health care initiatives.

The increasing sophistication of insurance mechanisms and the use of ambulatory care services as a control mechanism on the use of all services have led to an increase in the degree of structure of the health care system over the past few years. This increasing structure has occurred primarily in the private, nongovernmental sector. Integration of services will focus largely on multiple, independently organized systems of care that are competitive with one another.

The diversity of services, providers, and facilities involved in ambulatory care today is truly amazing and growing all the time. Many of these services and organizations are discussed in this chapter. Particular attention is directed toward rapidly expanding and innovative settings, such as group practice, and integration of settings and services through organized systems of care, especially in managed care.

Levels of Ambulatory Care Services

Ambulatory care services can be differentiated into a number of distinct levels or types of care. Primary prevention seeks to reduce the risks of illness or morbidity by removing or reducing disease-causing agents and opportunities for infection from our society. These activities include efforts to eliminate environmental pollutants that are suspected to cause diseases such as cancer. Other examples of primary prevention include encouraging people to use automobile seat belts, treatment of water and sewage, and sanitation inspections in restaurants. Preventive health services are more direct personal interventions to detect and prevent disease. Examples of these services include hypertension, diabetes, and cancer screening clinics and immunization programs. The combination of primary prevention and preventive services is our first line of defense against disease.

Medical care that is oriented toward the daily, routine needs of patients, such as initial diagnosis and continuing treatment of common illness, is termed *primary care*. This care is not highly complex and generally does not require sophisticated technology and personnel. The image of the general practitioner of bygone days, traveling from house to house ministering to the sick, represents the traditional role of primary care, which is replaced in today's society by considerably more skilled practitioners in more complex facilities.

In addition to providing services directly, the primary care professional may, in some settings, serve the role of patient advisor, advocate, and system "gatekeeper." In this coordinating role, the provider refers patients to sources of specialized care, gives advice regarding various diagnoses and therapies, and provides continuing care for chronic conditions. In many organized systems of care, such as managed care programs, this role is very important in controlling costs, utilization, and the rational allocation of resources.

The evolution of technology and medicine's increasing ability to intervene in illness have led to greater specialization of health care services. These more specialized services, termed *secondary* and *tertiary* care, are provided in both ambulatory and inpatient settings. The content of secondary and tertiary care practices is usually more narrowly defined than that of the primary care provider. Subspecialists, who provide the bulk of secondary and tertiary care, also often require more complex equipment and more highly trained support personnel than do primary care providers.

In recent years, the evolution of health care services has led to greatly expanded provision of secondary care on an outpatient, or ambulatory care, basis. Numerous surgical services of increasing complexity have been shifted to the ambulatory arena; recent advances in the use of fiber optic and other technologies suggest that this trend will continue. Diagnostic and therapeutic procedures that used to require hospitalization are also increasingly being performed in ambulatory settings.

There are no clear dividing lines for primary versus secondary and secondary versus tertiary care. Secondary services include "routine" hospitalization and specialized outpatient care. These services are more complex than those of primary care and include many diagnostic procedures as well as more complex therapies. Tertiary care includes the most complex services, such as open heart surgery, burn treatment, and transplantation, and is provided in inpatient hospital facilities.

SETTINGS FOR THE PROVISION OF AMBULATORY CARE

Use of Ambulatory Care Services

Historically, and at the present time, most ambulatory care services are provided in solo and group practice, office-based settings. Institutional settings for care, primarily the hospital, although an important component of the health care system, remain less prominent. Overlap between office-based practice and institutional settings is increasingly common, however, as the dividing lines between various components of the health care system continue to blur. Managed care programs especially tend to integrate these services.

An indication of the use and sites of ambulatory care visits is contained in Tables 4.1 and 4.2, which present survey results on utilization patterns, based on national data that are representative of the entire United States population. These data are taken from the National Health Interview Survey, a national survey of Americans' use of health care services, and they complement the utilization data presented in previous chapters.

Table 4.1 describes the number of physician contacts experienced by Americans in various sex and age categories as well as for family income and geographic regions. The very young and the very old report higher utilization of ambulatory services, and females, depending on age, generally experience higher utilization than males. The lowest income groups in our population, not coincidentally those of lower health status as well, experience the highest utilization of ambulatory services when the data are examined by income groups. In examining the data (not shown) by geographic regions, ambulatory services utilization is highest in those areas where managed care is most prevalent, particularly the West and Midwest regions of the country. Examining these data by place of contact

Table 4.1. Health Care Visits to Doctors' Offices, Emergency Departments, and Home Visits Within the Past 12 Months: United States, 2001

Characteristic	Number of Health Care Visits			
	None	One to Three Visits	Four to Nine Visits	Ten or More Visits
All persons	16.5	45.8	24.4	13.3
Age				
Under 18 years	11.6	54.6	26.1	7.6
Under 6 years	5.5	45.8	37.9	10.8
18–44 years	23.3	46.1	18.9	11.8
45–64 years	15.6	42.9	25.7	15.9
65 years and over	7.1	32.3	35.6	25.0
Sex				
Male	21.3	46.5	21.6	10.7
Female	11.9	45.1	27.1	15.9
Race				
White only	15.9	45.7	24.8	13.5
Black or African American only	16.4	46.4	24.0	13.2
American Indian and Alaska Native only	21.4	36.4	25.4	16.9
Asian only	20.8	48.3	22.3	8.6
Health Insurance Status				
Under 65 years of age				
Insured	14.1	49.1	24.2	12.6
Uninsured	37.5	41.4	14.6	6.5

reflects higher utilization of hospital outpatient departments by minorities and by those individuals with lower incomes. Relatively little care, except in the oldest age groups, is provided in patients' homes, quite a contrast from years gone by.

Use of Office Setting Services

Most utilization data are available from survey research results. To obtain more detailed information on health care use in physician office settings, the federal government has conducted periodic surveys of private, office-based physicians—the National Ambulatory Medical Care Survey. This survey involves a random sample of the nation's office-based, nonfederal physicians. Physicians are asked to complete a data collection form for each patient treated during a two-week interval.

Table 4.2 lists the most common reasons for all office visits. The relative prominence of routine care, of follow-up or ongoing care, and of relatively simple primary care is rather striking and reflects the predominance of "routine," day-to-day needs of patients seeking ambulatory care services.

Further understanding of the nature of the visits is obtainable from additional data regarding the services provided to patients and the interactions shared between patients and physicians. The drugs prescribed during the physician office visits are classified in Table 4.3. The most prevalent categories of drugs include cardiovascular and pain-relief agents. As technology changes, the classification distribution of various drug categories will likely change in prevalence as well.

Table 4.4 presents the distribution of office visits by the duration of the visit. Relatively few visits require either very short or very long physician contacts. The typical physician office visit requires only about 5 to 30 minutes of time. A high percentage of visits concluded with the recommendation that the patient return at a specified time interval for a follow-up visit. The

Table 4.2. Number and Percentage Distribution of Office Visits by the 20 Principal Reasons Most Frequently Mentioned by Patients, According to Patient's Sex: United States, 2001

Principal Reason for Visit	Number of Visits in Thousands	Patient's Sex (Percentage Distribution) Female	Male
All visits	880,487	100.0	100.0
General medical examination	68,844	7.4	8.5
Progress visit, not otherwise specified	39,783	4.4	4.7
Cough	27,062	2.7	3.6
Postoperative visit	23,995	2.9	2.5
Routine prenatal examination	19,848	3.8	—
Medication, other and unspecified kinds	16,457	1.9	1.8
Symptoms referable to throat	15,082	1.8	1.5
Back symptoms	13,707	1.5	1.7
Stomach pain, cramps, and spasms	13,594	1.6	1.5
Vision dysfunctions	13,555	1.5	1.6
Knee symptoms	12,743	1.4	1.5
Diabetes mellitus	12,502	1.1	1.9
Well-baby examination	12,361	1.2	1.7
Skin rash	12,088	1.3	1.5
Fever	10,910	1.0	1.5
Gynecological examination	10,782	2.1	—
Hypertension	10,467	1.1	1.3
Headache, pain in head	9,876	1.2	1.0
Nasal congestion	9,592	0.9	1.4
Earache or ear infection	9,449	1.2	0.9
All other reasons	517,791	57.8	60.2

SOURCE: *National Ambulatory Medical Care Survey: 2001 Summary* (Advance data from vital and health statistics; No. 337), D. K. Cherry, C. W. Burt, D. A. Woodwell, 2003; Hyattsville, MD: National Center for Health Statistics.

National Ambulatory Medical Care Survey thus provides valuable insight into the nature of office-based ambulatory care.

Table 4.3. Number and Percentage Distribution of Drug Mentions by Therapeutic Classification: United States, 2001

Therapeutic Classification	Number of Drug Mentions in Thousands	Percentage Distribution
All drug mentions	1,313,786	100.0
Cardiovascular-renal drugs	192,842	14.7
Drugs used for relief of pain	159,065	12.1
Respiratory tract drugs	152,952	11.6
Hormones and agents affecting hormonal mechanisms	142,513	10.8
Central nervous system drugs	114,059	8.7
Antimicrobial agents	113,969	8.7
Metabolic/nutrients	107,764	8.2
Skin/mucous membrane drugs	61,944	4.7
Gastrointestinal agents	58,033	4.4
Immunologics	52,595	4.0
Ophthalmics	39,169	3.0
Neurologics	33,565	2.6
Hermatologics	22,306	1.7
Anesthetic drugs	10,085	0.8
Oncolytic agents	7,211	0.5
Antiparasitics	5,631	0.4
Otologics	4,979	0.4
Contrast media/ radiopharmaceuticals	392	0.0
Other and unclassified	34,713	2.6

SOURCE: *National Ambulatory Medical Care Survey: 2001 Summary* (Advance data from vital and health statistics; No. 337), D. K. Cherry, C. W. Burt, D. A. Woodwell, 2003; Hyattsville, MD: National Center for Health Statistics.

Table 4.4. Number and Percentage Distribution of Office Visits by Duration of Visit: United States, 2001

Duration	Number of Visits in Thousands	Percentage Distribution
All visits	880,487	100.0
Visits at which no physician was seen	37,122	4.2
Visits at which a physician was seen	843,364	95.8
Total	843,364	100.0
1–5 minutes	34,424	4.1
6–10 minutes	167,627	19.9
11–15 minutes	316,998	37.6
16–30 minutes	266,933	31.7
31–60 minutes	54,426	6.5
61 minutes and over	2,956	0.4

SOURCE: *National Ambulatory Medical Care Survey: 2001 Summary* (Advance data from vital and health statistics; No. 337), D. K. Cherry, C. W. Burt, D. A. Woodwell, 2003; Hyattsville, MD: National Center for Health Statistics.

AMBULATORY PRACTICE SETTINGS

Significant differences exist among physician practice settings, and these are discussed in the following sections of this chapter. The two primary noninstitutional settings for the provision of ambulatory care are solo and group practice. Each of these settings may be a component of larger systems of care through such integrating mechanisms as referral arrangements, insurance contracts, and direct ownership of practices. An organized system of care can, in turn, be comprised of various settings or types of ambulatory care providers.

Although the solo practice of medicine has traditionally attracted the greatest number of practitioners, group practice and institutionally based services are now expanding dramatically, continuing a trend that has been building over the past 30 years. Changing lifestyles, the cost of establishing a practice, personal financial pressures on practitioners, contracting and affiliation opportunities under managed care, and the burdens of running a business have enhanced the attractiveness of group practice for many physicians. With sharp increases in the number of physicians beginning practice, the growth of alternative settings, and especially of group practice, has been dramatic. Although solo practice remains an important avenue for providing ambulatory care services, these other settings have rapidly assumed a more prominent and visible role, particularly as they provide a further mechanism for the integration, management, and control of health care services.

Solo Practice

Solo practitioners are difficult to characterize in a uniform way. Early sociological studies focused on specific questions, such as referral patterns or quality of care, and they did not provide a comprehensive picture of what the solo practitioner does. The studies that did contribute to a more complete understanding of the activities of solo practitioners were based on physicians in one geographic area or a particular specialty, and the results of these studies, although interesting and useful, may not be applicable to other practices or areas. In addition, solo practitioners are heterogeneous; they include many types of health care professionals who provide an immense array of services.

Some solo practitioners are subspecialists who provide secondary care primarily on referral from primary care practitioners. Under managed care, these subspecialists are being squeezed by reduced payment for specialty services, by capitation payment for population coverage, and by the increasing trend for gatekeepers to perform services that otherwise might have been referred to subspecialists. Some subspecialists provide both primary and secondary care, since they have insufficient work in their own specialties to achieve desired income levels.

Many solo practitioners, including those trained in general and family practice, internal medicine, pediatrics, and obstetrics and gynecology, provide primary care services, which has led to some controversy concerning which specialists should be providing primary care. Family medicine practitioners, in particular, complete with general internists in providing adult primary care and with pediatricians in providing child care, although the role of family practice is now firmly established, especially in managed care.

Most solo practitioners perform a number of functions in the office, including patient care, consultations, and administration and supervision of office staff. The requirements for administration and for supervision of personnel have been increasing in recent years. Solo practitioners are increasingly affiliating with managed care networks that help ensure a viable patient population.

Solo practice is often associated with an increased perception that the provider cares about the welfare of the patient, possibly resulting in a stronger patient-provider relationship than develops in other settings. There is some evidence that this situation, where it occurs, is a result of the lower level of bureaucracy or organizational complexity in solo practice. Because there is also some evidence that the relationship between patient and physician is related to patient compliance with medical regimens, patients who believe that they are receiving more personalized care may respond to the care process more positively.

Solo practitioners may not be as restricted in referrals to specialists as providers in some other settings, such as group practice, where organizational loyalties intervene. Managed-care contracts, however, may severely limit referral options.

The solo practitioner may feel a greater identification with the community served, since there is a more direct relationship between patient and provider. Organizational forms, especially managed care, that incorporate solo practitioners into larger systems of care may be decreasing some of this physician-patient bond, especially as providers are forced to discount fees, increase productivity, and focus on the cost-effectiveness of their practices.

From the provider's perspective, solo practice offers an opportunity to avoid organizational dependence and to be self employed; there is also no need to share resources or income with other providers. Philosophically, solo practice is most closely aligned with the traditional economic and political organizations that have characterized medicine; younger physicians faced with discounting, contracting, and networks for care, however, may no longer identify with the more traditional perspectives.

All of the increasingly complex problems of administering a practice must be dealt with in solo practice unless a professional manager is hired. Furthermore, competitive pressures in the health care industry are leading many practitioners to question the feasibility and desirability of going it alone. Many solo practitioners are now affiliated with larger entities such as independent practice associations, practice management companies, and other organizations. Thus solo practice offers distinct opportunities and has philosophical and emotional appeal but is far from devoid of problems and constraints, especially in light of the realities of medical practice today.

Group Practice

Office-based practice includes, in addition to solo practice, group practice. This form of practice has been growing in popularity in recent years, especially as the increasing pressures of practice have led many providers to seek alternative settings in which to work.

Group practice is an affiliation of three or more providers, usually physicians, who share income, expenses, facilities, equipment, medical records, and support personnel in the provision of services through a formal, legally constituted organization. The formal definition of group practice, developed by the American Medical Association and the Medical Group Management Association, is three

or more physicians formally organized to provide medical care, consultation, diagnosis, and/or treatment through the joint use of equipment and personnel, and with income from medical practice distributed in accordance with methods previously determined by members of the group. Although definitions of a group practice vary somewhat, the essential element is formal sharing of resources and income.

Traditionally, group practice has meant participation and ownership by physicians. Increasingly, however, as new and more diversified models for the provision of services are developed, other practitioners will participate in group practices. In some communities, for example, group practices of nurse practitioners may be the only sources of health services. Dentists, optometrists, podiatrists, and other specialized personnel are also increasingly organizing group practices.

History of Group Practice

Some of the earliest group practices in the United States were started by companies that needed to provide care to employees in rural sites where medical care was unobtainable. For example, the Northern Pacific Railroad organized a practice in 1883 to provide care to employees building the transcontinental railroad. This industrial clinic was one of a number of such clinics founded in the nineteenth century.

Even more significant, however, was the establishment of the Mayo Clinic in Rochester, Minnesota—the first successful nonindustrial group practice. The Mayo Clinic, originally organized as a single-specialty group practice in 1887 and later broadened into a multispecialty group, demonstrated that group practice was feasible in the private sector. The Mayo Clinic also represented a reputable model for group practice in a national atmosphere of fierce independence in which group practice was viewed with skepticism and distrust.

In 1932 a national committee, the Committee on the Costs of Medical Care, was established to assess health care needs for the nation. It issued a report that suggested a major role for group practice in the provision of medical care. The committee recommended that these groups be associated with hospitals to provide comprehensive care and that there be prepayment for all services.

Other constituencies, including some unions, also developed group practices. After World War II, a number of pioneering groups were established. In New York City, the Health Insurance Plan of New York was organized to provide prepaid medical care to the employees of the city—an idea promoted by Mayor Fiorello LaGuardia. On the West Coast, the Kaiser Foundation Health Plan was established to provide health care to employees of Kaiser Industries; Kaiser is an affiliation of plans and providers that is now serving millions of Americans across the nation. In Seattle, a revolutionary development included the establishment of Group Health Cooperative of Puget Sound, a consumer-owned cooperative prepaid group practice. It was founded by progressive individuals who were dissatisfied with the private medical care available to them in the late 1940s.

Developments in medical practice also spurred the group practice movement. Perhaps most notable was the increasing specialization of medicine and the rapid expansion of technology. This increasing sophistication meant that no individual practitioner could provide all the expertise that patients would require. It also meant that more complex and expensive facilities, equipment, and personnel were needed to care for patients.

Group practice provided a formal structure for sharing these costs among providers. Many people believed that resources would be used more efficiently in groups. In addition, multispecialty groups, encompassing more than one field, could provide patients with more of their health care under one roof and hence reduce problems of physical access to care and coordination of services.

Group practice was also thought to promote higher-quality care, since most of the different specialists whom a person required would be practic-

ing together and would thus have the opportunity to discuss patient problems among themselves, share a common medical record, and be more able to ensure the quality and continuity of care. Therefore, group practice was viewed by many as being advantageous for the physician—offering opportunities such as easily developed referral arrangements, sharing of after-hours coverage, greater flexibility in working hours, and less financial risk—while also benefiting the patient.

At times, opposition to group practice has occurred, mostly for political and philosophical reasons. The American Medical Association and local medical societies have on occasion raised objections to group practice. Many early group practices experienced difficulties when physicians were denied admitting privileges in local hospitals. Community-based specialists sometimes refused to treat patients referred by group practice physicians. Eventually, however, opposition to group practice lessened dramatically, and restrictive laws were challenged. The need to form affiliations for contracting under reimbursement programs and for achieving efficiencies in organizing health services more generally has strengthened the role of group practice.

Survey of Group Practice

The American Medical Association has conducted surveys of physician-oriented medical group practices in the United States on a periodic basis since 1965. These surveys represent the most comprehensive data available concerning the growth and characteristics of group practice in this country. Group practices that qualified within the American Medical Association's definition were identified from a variety of data sources and were then surveyed through a mail data collection instrument. The dramatic increase in popularity of practices is reflected in Table 4.5. Even more dramatic is the growth in the number of physicians in a group-practice setting. A higher percentage of all physicians in group practice work in multispecialty-oriented groups as compared to the percentage of

Table 4.5. Number of Medical Groups and Number of Physicians in Group Practice: United States, Selected Years

Year	Total Number of Groups	Number of Physician Positions in Group Practice
1969	6,371	40,093
1975	8,488	66,842
1980	10,762	88,290
1984	15,186	139,127
1988	16,495	155,628
1991	16,576	184,358
1995	19,787	210,811
1996	19,820	206,557
2003 (est.)	20,000–25,000	210,000–250,000

SOURCE: Adapted from *Medical Groups in the U.S., 1999 Edition. A Survey of Practice Characteristics*, by P. L. Havlicek, 1999; Chicago: American Medical Association, and estimate.

total groups that are multispecialty, largely because the average multispecialty group is substantially larger than the average single-specialty group.

Specialty distribution of physicians in group practice has not changed dramatically in recent years. The specialties that account for the largest percentage of physicians participating in group practice include family and general practice, internal medicine, anesthesiology, obstetrics and gynecology, pediatrics, and radiology; many groups are now involved in managed care contracting.

Relatively few groups account for a significant percentage of all physicians in group practice as presented in Table 4.6. As would be expected, most of the larger groups are multispecialty, while the smaller groups are predominantly single specialty. The geographic distribution of group practice in the United States is dominated by seven states, which account for 40 percent of all groups. These states are California, Pennsylvania, New York, Texas, Illinois, Florida, and Ohio.

Interestingly, nearly all larger groups employ an administrator. The market for trained group-practice administrators has grown substantially over the past few years, and its growth is likely to continue as the number of group practices increases.

New Forms of Group Practice

Managed care has led to the development of new forms of group practice to allow physicians alternative settings in which to participate in contracting arrangements such as the independent practice associations (IPAs). Most of this innovation is the result of the need to form contractual arrangements with health systems, managed care organizations, and insurers. These new organizational forms are continuing to evolve. Smaller practices, in particular, have needed to seek out alliances that facilitate contractual arrangements under managed care. Smaller practices face disadvantages with regard to availability of capital investment, professional management, and often overhead and other costs.

Table 4.6. Total Groups and Group Physician Positions by Size of Group, 1996

Size of Group	Groups		Group Physician Positions	
	Percent	Number	Percent	Number
3–4	45.9	8,938	15.0	30,978
5–6	22.9	4,451	11.7	24,096
7–9	12.6	2,449	9.2	19,052
10–15	8.8	1,713	9.9	20,350
16–25	4.8	937	8.8	18,484
26–49	2.7	535	9.1	18,815
50–99	1.2	228	7.5	15,603
100 or more	1.1	218	28.7	59,179

SOURCE: Adapted from *Medical Groups in the U.S., 1999 Edition. A Survey of Practice Characteristics*, by P. L. Havlicek, 1999; Chicago: American Medical Association.

Larger practices and new approaches to creating affiliations of groups facilitate potential economies of scale, efficiencies in management and operations, improved contracting potential and market involvement, and enhanced deployment of capital.

Group practices may be formed by or affiliated with larger organizations such as hospitals or health systems. Groups may be affiliated with one another through various mechanisms that may provide management services and contracting potential for solo and smaller group practitioners while preserving a degree of independence for these practitioners. There are for-profit management companies and some not-for-profit entities providing services to physician groups and, in some instances, actually purchasing groups outright, as well.

From a pragmatic point of view, many of these new forms of group practice are designed to facilitate the participation of solo- and group-practice physicians in the rapidly changing world of managed care where practices must be managed efficiently and have easy access to contracting mechanisms. Key issues include physician autonomy and involvement in governance and management; sources and uses of capital investment; control over physician clinical practice patterns; extent of control by a larger entity over physician staff, facilities, and daily operation; and relationships with other entities such as hospitals, insurers, managed care organizations, and, of course, patients.

An Assessment of Group Practice

A critical assessment of group practice yields distinct advantages and disadvantages for both patients and providers as compared to other modalities for providing ambulatory services. Some of these are summarized in Table 4.7. Specific advantages and disadvantages vary from group to group. Some of the topics listed under patient or provider perspectives could readily pertain to both.

From the perspective of the provider, the advantages of group practice include shared operation of the practice; joint ownership of facilities and equipment; centralized administrative functions; and, in larger groups, a professional manager. The professional manager can provide expertise in areas often lacking among the providers such as billing; personnel management; patient scheduling; ordering of supplies; and, recently, of particular importance, negotiating, contracting, and related matters.

Financially, the group relieves the provider of the heavy initial investment often required to establish a practice. In most groups, however, co-ownership requires that new members buy into the group through purchase of a share of the group's capital over a period of time.

The burden of operating costs is also lessened for any individual member of a group. Rather than having to independently absorb the ups and downs of a practice, as do solo practitioners, those involved in a group practice share the income and expenses within the group, allowing for moderation of those fluctuations experienced in individual practices. For example, a solo practitioner who becomes ill may have no practice income aside from disability insurance, whereas a group member's income may continue during a short period of illness, since other providers are simultaneously generating revenue.

The participation of physicians in group practice also has a significant advantage in facilitating the development of arrangements for contracting and negotiating. Even single-specialty groups, with shared on-call services and subspecialization of group members, are able to offer more to the market on a contractual basis than the individual practitioner. Having a professional manager to negotiate on behalf of the group further enhances the relative attractiveness of group practice, particularly for physicians who lack experience in interpreting and negotiating contracts.

Patient care responsibilities are also shared in group practice. This sharing results in greater flexibility of working hours for the provider, as well as more time for vacation and continuing education, without sacrificing the quality of care for the patient.

Table 4.7. Some Advantages and Disadvantages of Group Practice[a]

Advantages	Disadvantages
From the perspective of the provider	
Availability of professional manager	Less individual freedom
Organizational responsibility for patient	Possible excessive use of specialists
Less physician administrative time	Fewer outside consultants
Shared capital expense	Possible reduced identification with patient and community
Shared financial risk	Group rather than individual decision making
Improved contracting and negotiating ability	Sharing of all problems
Better coverage and shared on-call shifts	Necessity of working with others
More flexible working hours	Less individual incentive and more orientation toward security
More peer interaction	Income limitations
Increased access to specialists	Income distribution arguments
Broader array of ancillary services	
Stable income for providers	
No direct financial concerns with patients	
Lower initial investment	
More time for continuing education	
More flexible vacation time	
Generally excellent benefits	
Possible efficiencies of scale	
Use of nonphysician practitioners	
Managed care contracting efficiency	
From the perspective of the patient	
Care under one roof	Possible lessening of provider–patient relationship
Availability of specialists, laboratories, and so on	Possible overuse of ancillary services
Improved coverage and emergency care	Possible high provider turnover
Central location of medical and administrative records	Heavy patient loads and possible increase in waiting time
Simplified referrals	Less provider incentive for care
Peer interaction among providers	More bureaucracy
Better administration of group	
Possible promotion of efficiency in patient care	
Possible improved quality monitoring/standards	

[a] Some advantages and disadvantages could be included under both provider and patient categories.

Sharing of patient care may have some other potential benefits. These include more peer interaction as a result of informal discussions and referral of patients among providers. The inclusion of more providers also results in the availability, by necessity, of a wider range of specialists and ancillary services, which represents a convenience for both providers and patients as well as a source of added revenue for the group.

Does the sharing of administrative and patient care activities within group practice result in better care at lower cost? The evidence is mixed. Many people believe that effective group management uses resources more efficiently than solo practice, but others question this view. More analytical research indicates some economies of scale, or efficiencies, attributable to the grouping of resources for smaller groups, but possibly less so for larger and more bureaucratic groups. The use of personnel may be more advantageous in group than in solo practice. Receptionists, medical records specialists, laboratory and radiology technicians, nurses, and other personnel may be used more efficiently and in the specialized areas of their training in many medium- and larger-sized groups. In addition, there is some question about whether any savings that are achieved will be returned to consumers or insurers or simply represent higher income for providers. Further, the increasing supply of physicians may reduce the desirability of employing mid-level practitioners, except in certain managed care settings.

The effect of groups on patient care, especially on the quality of care, is an important issue. Sharing of medical records, peer interaction, easy referrals and consultations with specialists, more sophisticated and accessible ancillary services, and more skilled and diversified support personnel are all arguments suggested in support of higher-quality care in group practice. Pressures from managed-care contracts, however, may affect quality-related issues such as use, access, and appropriateness of care.

Group practice also offers advantages to patients and their communities. For the patient, the group offers a wide range of services under one roof so that travel between providers is reduced and access increased. A unified medical record can contribute to continuity of care and less duplication in diagnosis and treatment. Some groups also own or operate hospitals and thus further extend the integration and scope of the services that they provide, an especially important consideration in negotiating with employers and insurers.

Group practices usually offer more accessible care after normal working hours. Some groups also offer emergency services through their own emergency rooms or clinics. Groups with a broader community perspective may even be involved in programs such as school health services and community immunization efforts, and the use of a professional manager should benefit the patient through more efficient scheduling and patient flow and improved overall management of the practice.

There are also distinct disadvantages to group practice for providers, patients, and communities. From the perspective of the provider, practicing in a group implies less individual freedom, with a variety of restrictions imposed through the sharing of a practice. Ideologically, the limitations of a group in this regard may be difficult for some people to accept, since medicine has traditionally been an individualistic enterprise. In addition to reduced freedom, group practice entails sharing responsibilities and problems with others.

The financial advantages for group practice are a trade-off against some restrictions on income generation and the necessity of complying with the group's income distribution and practice pattern requirements. Thus, there often is more security and less risk but also less incentive and reward for individual initiative and production.

From a community perspective, groups may reduce the geographic dispersion of providers and thus increase difficulties of physical access to care. In addition, groups may reduce competition in the health care marketplace by consolidating what would otherwise be competing providers. Consolidation may eventually reduce the ability of insurers, employers, and other plan sponsors to negotiate favorable terms for contracted care.

The changing organizational structure of the health care system is also changing some aspects of the role of ambulatory care services from the perspectives of providers, consumers, and the community. Ambulatory care is assuming a much greater role in the rationing of care, especially for primary care, and in the control of referrals and use of specialty, laboratory, and other services. These changes are especially notable in managed care and for hospital-sponsored systems of care.

The financial and operational perspectives of managing a group practice have become much more complex in recent years as a result of changes in reimbursement, legal developments, expectations on the part of physicians and other providers, and payer and patient demands for accountability. Managed-care contracts in particular require increasing sophistication in reporting of data and in claims processing while government oversight and pressures for improved quality have raised the bar in internal organization information systems and evaluation efforts. With ambulatory care services increasingly assuming responsibility for patient care management and quality and costs accountability, more sophisticated information systems and monitoring mechanisms are constantly being introduced into the management of these organizations.

The implications of these structural changes in the provision of health care are profound. Consumers are affected in terms of where and how they receive services. Providers are affected by changes in their affiliations, referral patterns, incentives, and practice characteristics. And, finally, the community is obviously affected by the changing organization of services, by the formation of alliances, and by shifts in the economic and political clout of various providers.

INSTITUTIONALLY BASED AMBULATORY SERVICES

In addition to solo and group practice in the traditional private sector, many institutions have expanded their involvement in ambulatory care. These institutionally based settings, especially those associated with hospitals, are discussed next.

The hospital has evolved from an institution for poor people who could not be cared for at home to a provider of a full range of health services from primary to tertiary care. As technological advances have brought more services into the hospital and expanded the scope of care provided, the hospital has assumed an especially important role in the provision of highly complex health services. At the same time, an increasing number of people have sought primary care from hospitals, sometimes as a result of lack of access to other sources of care.

Outpatient and Ambulatory Care Clinics

The increased demands placed on hospitals for care taxed the ability of many facilities to respond with appropriate and adequate resources. The result was overcrowded facilities; the wrong mix of services, equipment, and personnel to respond to patient needs; and extremely dissatisfied consumers and providers. Most hospitals have now successfully responded to these demands by expanding outpatient services and hiring full-time providers to staff redesigned hospital ambulatory facilities.

Traditional hospital outpatient services have been provided in clinics and emergency rooms. In many hospitals, clinics once had second-class status as compared to complex and expensive inpatient services. However, as hospitals are increasingly recognizing the important role of primary care, especially in managed care contracting, and are seeking to expand the base of patients who are potential users of inpatient and ancillary services, more attention is being directed toward improving clinic operations and services.

Hospital clinics include both primary care and specialty clinics. Many hospitals differentiate between clinics for walk-in patients without appointments and those for scheduled visits. Specialty clinics are usually organized by department and provide services such as ophthalmology, neurology, and allergy care. In teaching hospitals, clinics serve as important settings in which house staff members provide ongoing care to patients and follow-up after hospitalization. Increasingly, clinics also provide an opportunity to expose medical students and house staff to ambulatory care services in order to complement the traditionally more extensive experience with inpatient care. With the increasing role of ambulatory care in health services, this trend is significant.

Many hospital primary-care clinics evolved from an orientation of service to the poor and were staffed by physicians who served without reimbursement in exchange for staff privileges. The level of commitment to the patient under such circumstances was—not surprisingly—less than desirable. Many hospitals now employ physicians and other practitioners as full-time clinic staff. Some hospitals have established primary-care group practices to complement other outpatient services and to assume the burden of providing primary care to patients who seek most of their health care from the hospital.

The development of a group practice has advantages for both consumers and the hospital by providing comprehensive and accessible care and by removing primary care patients from facilities that are not designed to serve their needs, such as emergency rooms. Development of these group practices also has the potential of increasing use of the hospital's inpatient and ancillary services, an advantage if occupancy is low. Hospitals with ambulatory care resources can negotiate contracts for providing a wide range of both inpatient and outpatient services. They are subsequently also able to more effectively control the use of services and thus costs.

Questions have been raised, however, concerning the ability of hospitals to compete effectively in an arena in which they have not been overly successful in the past. But the increasingly competitive nature of the hospital and the health care marketplace is forcing many hospitals to enter this area of practice even if they are uncertain about doing so.

Ambulatory Surgery Centers

A further innovation in hospital-based care has been the development of ambulatory surgery centers.

Originating in hospitals in Washington, D.C., Los Angeles, and elsewhere, these organized hospital units provide one-day surgical care. Patients are usually screened for acceptability by their personal surgeons and then report at an assigned date and time for surgery. The surgeon is supported by the unit's facilities, equipment, and personnel, and the patient is discharged 1 to 3 hours after surgery when recovery from anesthesia is sufficiently complete.

In the early 1970s, freestanding ambulatory surgery centers were opened; one of the first was in Phoenix, Arizona. These facilities are independent of hospitals and usually provide a full range of services for the types of surgery that can be performed on an outpatient basis. Community surgeons are granted operating privileges and can perform surgery in these facilities when the patient agrees and when there are no medical contraindications.

Other facilities are also used for ambulatory or outpatient surgery. Many physicians traditionally performed surgery in their offices, although this practice has declined in some specialties as a result of malpractice concerns and the increasing availability of better-equipped and -staffed alternative facilities. Some specialties, such as oral surgery, plastic surgery, and ophthalmology, extensively use office-based facilities.

Freestanding emergency centers have also opened in some cities, paralleling the success of ambulatory surgery centers. In addition to responding to urgent problems, they sometimes provide a wide range of primary care. The future of specialized ambulatory centers, both in hospitals and as freestanding facilities, will probably include further expansion into other areas of health care, ranging from sports medicine to women's health care.

Even greater innovation has occurred in recent years. Freestanding postsurgical recovery centers for short nonhospital stays of 1 to 3 nights are available to provide a less intensive recovery setting for less complex surgical cases. Mobile diagnostic facilities with sophisticated imaging equipment have been operational for a number of years. Even mobile physician vans, in a return to the house call, now transport the physician along with his/her office to the patient's home without sacrificing technological capabilities. The Internet is used for patient education, scheduling, communication, and other purposes. Remote monitoring and other advanced applications are under development as well. The challenge for the future remains to identify economically feasible and innovative approaches to providing patient care that expedite the care process and are accepted by consumers, providers, and payers.

Emergency Rooms

The emergency room, like other hospital departments, has undergone transformation in recent years. The emergency room has expanded in the range of services offered and in complexity. An especially important long-term trend has been the increasing use of the emergency room for primary care. Since the emergency room requires sophisticated facilities and highly trained personnel and must be accessible 24 hours a day, costs are high and services are not designed for nonurgent care. To reduce the burden on the emergency room and to meet patient need more effectively, many hospitals treat patients on a triage basis. In this process, often performed by a nurse, the patient's health care needs are determined and the patient is referred to a more appropriate source of care within the hospital. Misuse of the emergency room has received considerable attention over the past 30 years.

Emergency medical services have also been increasingly integrated with other community resources. Included are drug and alcohol abuse treatment programs, mental health centers, and voluntary agencies. Most major urban centers have developed formal emergency medical systems that incorporate all hospital emergency rooms as well as transportation and communication systems. In these communities, people needing emergency care either transport themselves or call an emergency number (such as 911). An ambulance is dispatched

by a central communications center that also identifies and alerts the most appropriately equipped and located hospital. In many communities, regional hospital-based trauma centers have been built with extremely sophisticated capabilities. Specialized ambulance services, including mobile coronary care units and shock-trauma vans, are also increasingly prevalent.

GOVERNMENT PROGRAMS

In addition to private sector and institutionally initiated efforts, government programs have been designed to increase the availability of health care resources in many communities. These programs have adapted some of the concepts of private institutional settings, especially those of group practice.

Neighborhood health centers were funded starting in 1965 as part of the War on Poverty under the Economic Opportunity Act, and in the 1970s through the Public Health Service. Originally intended to serve approximately 25 million people, this federal program never reached its initial objectives. It was designed to provide primary medical care with a family orientation and was targeted for population groups in need of services, as reflected by such indicators as disease prevalence and income level. At the same time, the centers were intended to employ people from the communities they served in positions that would offer opportunities for training and advancement. Responsiveness to community needs was to be ensured by a board or advisory panel. The centers were to recognize that the broad attributes of a community, such as housing and employment, contributed to health and illness.

Although these health centers were originally intended to serve the poor, changes in federal policy that encouraged them to collect fees from patients and from third-party insurers have broadened the socioeconomic mixture of patients obtaining care. However, the centers still predominantly serve the medically indigent. Sources of funding have been broadened to include local government as well. Pressures for achieving self-sufficiency have been very powerful in recent years.

A related category of provider, the free clinic, evolved from a strong social commitment but has had to face similar financial realities. The combination of former free clinics, neighborhood health centers, public agency clinics, and some hospital clinics and groups now forms an informal safety net of providers for individuals who lack private insurance or access to other sources of care, or who simply need care from an available, sympathetic provider. Many of these providers now contract on their own or in coalitions with other providers to make care accessible to various individuals under government entitlement programs and sometimes in managed care arrangements as well.

Other community health centers that have been funded by the federal government include migrant health centers serving transient farm workers in agricultural areas and rural health centers. The National Health Service Corps supported practitioners who were placed in urban and rural areas with shortages of medical resources. Other innovations, such as mobile health vans in rural areas, have also been used to expand the scope of services. The Community Mental Health Center program was established to provide ambulatory mental health services in underserved areas. Community Mental Health Centers were intended to provide outpatient services and emergency care and to work with other community agencies to foster action and concern for mental health.

In recent years, community health centers have evolved into larger practices with multiple sources of support, including increasing reliance on patient fees and private donations and updated federal legislation and support. Many of these centers have become more businesslike in their operations. Yet most still face serious problems in attracting adequate financing, in attracting and retaining physicians, and in diversifying their patient mix, especially with regard to patients with insurance or the ability to pay for services on their own. The

shift of funding for entitlement programs to prepaid contracts may provide more financial stability for some of these providers in the future. Conflicts exist in some centers over the historical mission of serving the medically indigent versus the need for enhanced fiscal diversity and adopting a more business-oriented approach to operations.

The federal government, in addition to supporting a variety of community-based health services organizations, directly operates many health facilities. The Veterans Administration includes the largest health services system under a unified management structure in the United States, with 163 hospitals and many clinics. This system provides needed care to millions of veterans throughout the nation. The military services also provide health care to millions of individuals in the armed forces and have developed extensive regionalized facilities throughout the world.

The Gulf War, combined with the war against terrorism and the war in Iraq, increasingly stressed capacity of both the Veterans Administration and the military health care delivery systems. Congressional action in the mid-1990s increasing the scope of eligibility for veterans benefits and the legacy of previous conflicts has also created far greater potential demand for services, especially for the Veterans Administration system. The aging of the military veteran population has and will increasingly cause demand for health care and long-term care services for the foreseeable future. The Veterans Administration, in particular, has tried to improve its operations and scope of services to respond to this increasing demand, but financial support for the Veterans Administration mission has thus far been inadequate to meet these demands.

Government has a special responsibility for providing health care to a number of groups within the country. The Indian Health Service is charged with ensuring access to medical care on Indian reservations and in certain other locations. Although the difficulties of operating a largely rural system are immense, the Indian Health Service has succeeded in bringing modern medicine to many people.

NONINSTITUTIONAL HEALTH SERVICES

As noted in the introduction to this chapter, there are many ways in which ambulatory and community health services are provided. Although only the most prevalent types of provider and service are discussed here, each helps to meet the many health care needs of a community. The list is nearly endless, and a number of services warrant further discussion.

Home health services are provided by visiting nurse associations, proprietary companies, some hospitals, public health departments, and other agencies. These services allow people to remain in their homes and yet receive essential health services, thereby reducing costs and increasing the quality of life for many.

Rural health care has required unique and innovative solutions in many communities, especially in the absence of adequate supplies of physicians and facilities. In rural Alaska, many towns are served by physicians and other professionals who regularly fly in to treat patients. Satellites and the Internet are used to facilitate communications with specialists in urban medical centers, since even ordinary communications in remote areas may be difficult. Rural health care in many areas remains a challenging test of the ingenuity and resourcefulness of the health services system and community residents.

The Internet and more sophisticated imaging and computer systems have also greatly expanded the use of teleconferencing, remote imaging, and many other technologies related to health care delivery, and these are likely to continue to evolve in the future.

Other community health services not discussed in detail here include, but are not limited to, school health services; prison health services; vision care; dental care provided by solo, group, and institutionally based practitioners; foot care from podiatrists; and drug dispensing from pharmacists, who often also extensively advise and educate consumers. Voluntary agencies also provide health care services such as cancer screening clinics and health education. Finally, many indigenous health practitioners offer their services in this country and abroad. These practitioners include chiropractors, "medicine men," naturopaths, and others. The supportive and sometimes curative role of these individuals is often underestimated.

Among the most important contributions to reductions in mortality and morbidity in the twentieth century have been such public health measures as the improvement of sanitation, ensurance of potable water supplies, and upgraded housing. In recent years, there has also been an increased awareness of the need to control air and water pollution, to reduce exposure to carcinogens, and to improve and ensure the quality of the environment. The contribution of these efforts to health far exceeds, dollar for dollar, efforts to treat illness once it occurs. Their importance to ambulatory care is mentioned here, however, because public health agencies have responsibility for a remarkable range of relevant services.

In this context, it is important to emphasize that health care and ambulatory care services also must successfully interact with other aspects of our society. These other areas include social and welfare services, accident prevention in industry and in transportation, protection of the environment, improvement of food and water supplies, and even the general economic well-being of society, as health is directly correlated with employment and income security.

ORGANIZATION OF AMBULATORY CARE SYSTEMS

The changing structure of the health services system has had tremendous implications for ambulatory care services. The increased movement toward integrated systems of care and managed care has led ambulatory care services to assume a central role in the design and operation of many insurance and delivery programs. In addition, those paying for health services, including employers and insurers, have increasingly focused attention on the role that ambulatory care services can provide in improving the coordination and control of care as well as in reducing costs through the reduction of duplication and the shifting of services to lower-cost settings.

Those organizations constructing large-scale, integrated systems of care are continuing to seek existing ambulatory care structures, or are building new ones, as a means to complete their systems. In particular, insurers, hospitals, and other organizational entities are developing or purchasing ambulatory care resources such as medical practices, clinics, and other existing networks. Government units, such as the military, have long recognized the key attributes of ambulatory care in coordinating and controlling the overall utilization of services and, then, the cost and quality of care. These trends are likely to continue.

Many key design attributes of ambulatory care are essential for both the effective operation of ambulatory services and for the full integration of these services into larger systems of care. Ambulatory care is important in providing access to care, particularly within larger integrated systems. Access considerations include scope of services provided and hours of operation as well as distribution of resources throughout a geographic region populated by the target group of consumers. Physical access to the facilities must also be assured, including such considerations as parking, access to public transportation where appropriate, and access to physician facilities for the handicapped.

The scope of services provided must respond to population needs. These needs differ depending on whether the population is enrolled through insurance or entitlement programs or fee-for-service. How the population is served differs substantially in each situation. For all situations, however, decisions must be made concerning the type of care to be provided on an ambulatory versus an inpatient basis.

Marketing advantages can be achieved in the ambulatory care setting by recognizing the special needs of consumers, such as having multilingual staff available where appropriate. The friendliness of the staff and the physical attractiveness of the facilities can have dramatic effects on patient attitudes and satisfaction, not only with the ambulatory care provider but in the larger system of care as well. Thus, ambulatory care provides an influential marketing function in any system of care. Ambulatory care services also generally provide an opportunity for educating the consumer in terms of both health behaviors and appropriate use of the system. This educational role can contribute to cost containment by having patients help in managing their use. Ambulatory care can provide a key role in the overall provision of coordinated and continuous care. By accepting the gatekeeper role of the primary care physician, using medical records and other administrative tracking of patients, and avoiding duplication of services and unnecessary care, the ambulatory care setting can contribute handsomely to the overall effectiveness of all care provided to the patient. Physician payment incentives can facilitate an enhanced coordinating role for ambulatory care. Centralization of responsibility for patient care thus must be clearly assigned.

Mechanisms for monitoring patient and provider behavior to ensure compliance with health system operating guidelines are essential. There is also evidence that more effective continuity of care is associated with higher levels of patient compliance regarding medical regimens, which, in turn, may lead to better health outcomes and eventually lower utilization rates. Patient satisfaction is generally greater when continuity and coordination of care are achieved—both effective marketing and cost-containment tools.

The quality of care should reflect not only adequate medical skills but also a caring attitude on the part of the provider. Consumers in ambulatory care are capable of detecting some aspects of the technical quality of care, but they are even more aware of provider and system attitudes and behavior. Responding to the consumer is increasingly important in the competitive environment.

AMBULATORY CARE AND THE CHALLENGE OF MANAGED CARE

Ambulatory care services have been and will continue to be dramatically affected by the evolution of managed care. Managed care serves to shift considerable risk to practitioners and forces greater efficiencies in the ambulatory care arena. Clinical responsibility in many ambulatory care practices not only for patient care but also for allocation of resources and broader aspects of clinical decision making have also been enhanced by the pressures of managed care. Since managed care is focused on controlling provider and patient behavior, most of that control is being exercised through the ambulatory care arena. These pressures have allowed ambulatory care providers to gain greater power within the health care system, but with enhanced power comes increased responsibility, risk, financial pressures, and frictions with providers, insurers, and patients. Increasingly, the shift of managed care toward organizational forms that are associated with greater controls over resources, providers, and patients is increasing the pressure on those involved in the provision of ambulatory care services. The move toward more integrated health care systems has decreased practitioner autonomy and imposed additional managerial controls and pressures on all participants.

The role of ambulatory care in controlling the patient, particularly through such mechanisms as gatekeepers and various forms of utilization control, places the provider in a more difficult position with regard to patient satisfaction and clinical decision making. Rationing, both directly and indirectly, may result from fiscal pressures and risk shifting under managed care and is exacerbating

these pressures. Practitioners in ambulatory care increasingly must face new realities regarding incentives for income and the quality and quantity of the patient's services. All of these changes are appreciably affecting the ambulatory care arena and its participants.

At the same time as the financial and clinical practice pressures build, competition in the health care marketplace is requiring ambulatory care practitioners to provide friendly but efficient care that is customer oriented in a manner that attracts the patient but also controls the resources.

Clinical and managerial information systems have gained increasing importance in ambulatory care. Fiscal reports that reflect costs, expenditures, and other financial indicators are important in light of risk shifting under managed care contracts. Clinical measures of performance are increasingly utilized to assess physician practice patterns and relative performance among physicians in multispecialty groups. Managed care organizations and insurers are also utilizing such data for economic credentialing and other assessments of not only clinical but also financial performance on the part of practitioners. These trends concern many observers, since access, utilization, quality, and rationing are all affected by use of resources and allocation of services.

A developing major trend in ambulatory care is the increasing role of consumers in both managing their own care processes and in accepting increased levels of responsibility for decision making and utilization. Consumers have access to an unprecedented level of sophisticated information related to health care, disease, and illness. In addition, technological applications on the part of provider organizations are increasingly facilitating the communication with patients through e-mail, Internet, Web pages, and other approaches to facilitate interaction with consumers. In some organizations, consumers can access individualized health-related information pertinent to their own illnesses and disease status. Preventive information and health promotion services are also frequently available through Internet resources and in other educational programs. The trend in managed care and other ambulatory care settings toward consumer-driven health services increasingly looks toward patients as at least partial partners in decision making and in accessing alternative interventions and therapies. Patient expectations have also been greatly enhanced by more sophisticated clientele and much greater access to biomedical and health-related information. At the same time, many insurance plans are attempting to facilitate this increased role for consumers in part in the expectation that resources will be utilized more appropriately and efficiently and that alternative sources of information may lead to decreased in-person delivery costs. Increasingly, the diffusion of technology related to computerized medical records, computerized laboratory results and radiology scans, and the availability of information on clinical trials and other state-of-the-art advances is facilitating patient and provider interaction as well as allowing patients increased access to alternative sources of therapy, to second opinions, and to many other resources within the nation's health care system. Finally, cultural patterns, alternative therapies such as herbal medicine, and even rumors are more readily available as a result of vast media and Internet pathways for the diffusion of information. The influence of these trends is clearly changing the relationship between provider and patient and the role of the patient in accessing, utilizing, and evaluating ambulatory health care and other services in the health care system.

The future of health services, particularly with the pressures inherent in managed care and technological advances, will be characterized by further shifts in services from inpatient to ambulatory care settings. Ambulatory care practices will need to respond with appropriate and innovative service delivery options including new equipment, technology, specialized personnel, and facilities. Competition will be driven in managed care

contracting in part by the ability to provide cost-effective care in more innovative and appropriate settings.

Affiliations of provider organizations ranging from direct ownership in integrated systems to loose confederations and affiliations developed through contractual arrangements will enhance integration, coordination, managerial efficiency, and provision of clinical services. All group practice, and even solo, practitioners must be prepared to participate in various forms of networks, integrated systems, coordinated service provider organizations, and other innovative approaches to organizing the health care delivery system.

In recent years, the intensity of the financial and delivery pressures placed on ambulatory care providers has increased still further. Managed care contracting has resulted in tremendous stress owing to increasingly cost-conscious negotiations on the part of payers and demands through contractual mechanisms for increased accountability and reporting from ambulatory care providers. Provider, and to an extent consumer, dissatisfaction with these arrangements and their inherent stresses is now leading to a backlash. In some instances, managed-care companies are beginning to back off of their demands for accountability and practice oversight. The trend toward increased provider practice flexibility and independence is starting to accelerate. However, increasing costs in the health care sector continue to erode the foundation for the financial and operational aspects of the relationships between ambulatory care providers and payers. The future of various ambulatory care settings and arrangements will continue to be dependent on payer arrangements that, in turn, are impacted by trends in health care costs, delivery mechanisms and technology, consumer preference and demands, and government and employer policy development.

The challenge in ambulatory care is to effectively shift from a traditionally reactive set of providers, attitudes, and operational approaches to the proactive leadership role needed in today's competitive environment. Ambulatory care once meant a largely unaffiliated and unstructured set of small providers responding as business walked in the door. Now ambulatory care is a key element in the structuring of large-scale systems. These systems require financial and contractual arrangements with providers, and these ties are critical to all concerned parties.

The system's structure itself vitally affects the role of ambulatory care services; ambulatory care can, in turn, be vital to the success of the system. In managed care systems, the ability to control providers and consumers—and hence costs— depends on structuring the system based on the controlling role of ambulatory care and performing needed services through ambulatory delivery vehicles where feasible, while also maintaining quality. Ideally, quality and access will maintain acceptable minimum levels under any delivery system, and controls will be built in to monitor both.

From a health care delivery perspective, as opposed to the financial focus of other chapters, the demands on ambulatory care to provide a marketing, integrating, controlling, and organizing function are great. At the same time, services must retain the attributes of high quality, meeting specific patient needs, and offering a stimulating and rewarding environment for the providers as well. This is no small challenge.

STUDY QUESTIONS

1. What services are included under the rubric of ambulatory care?
2. What is the role of prevention in the nation's health care system?
3. To what extent and in what ways can we change our lifestyles to reduce the need for health care services?
4. How has group practice expanded over the past 30 years, and what are its advantages and disadvantages?
5. How frequently and in which locations do Americans visit physicians, and what services do they obtain?
6. What are some recent innovations in the delivery of ambulatory health care services?

CHAPTER 5

Public Health Services

Chapter Objectives

1. To describe the role of preventive health services and public health.
2. To depict the history and nature of public health services in the United States.

Public health services include some ambulatory care services provided through clinics, as well as a broad array of prevention-related services, and other statutory responsibilities. Public health agencies at the state and local levels form the first line of defense against disease and illness and biological terrorism, in this country. Further support is provided at the federal level through the National Centers for Disease Control and Prevention as well as other agencies.

PUBLIC HEALTH SERVICES

Public health services had their origin in part in the prevention of the spread of infectious diseases. Epidemics of smallpox, bubonic plague, cholera, typhoid fever, venereal disease, malaria, tuberculosis, and other diseases have taken a terrible toll throughout history. Industrialization and the migration of population to urban areas increased the risk of infectious diseases.

The need for safe water and food supplies in urban areas created greater threats to life than were found in agricultural environments. Increasing modernization has also brought with it the diseases and epidemics of modern society, such as mental illness; chronic diseases including cancer, heart disease, and stroke; diseases associated with industrialization and work-site risks; and diseases of lifestyles, such as vehicular accidents and acquired immunodeficiency syndrome (AIDS).

By the late 1800s, many large and medium-sized communities had health departments. In large cities, the public health bureaucracies grew as the problems they faced multiplied. These problems included sanitation, protection of food, housing needs, and, of course, traditional functions such as vital statistics registration. Other problems, such as rodent control, also cropped up with industrialization and increasing urban density, while the spread of contagious diseases, such as tuberculosis and venereal disease, continued. Waves of immigration increased the density of population in many cities, and working conditions in factories and mills further exacerbated the problems of modern society.

By the turn of the century, the majority of states had health departments at the state level. State departments were also involved in communicable disease control, in the operation of state laboratories, in health education, and in the regulation of food and water supplies.

Federal involvement in public health expanded substantially after 1935, but various federal agencies were involved in public health even prior to this time. In the 1800s, the federal government operated the marine hospital service, which subsequently became the U.S. Public Health Service, with hospitals in various ports that focused on care for merchant seamen and on infectious disease control.

Federal responsibility in public health expanded greatly after the 1935 passage of the Social Security Act. In addition, the federal government became heavily involved in biomedical research with the expansion of the National Institutes of Health.

In recent years, the federal government has been much more proactive in the public health arena. Federal grants for a wide variety of categorical health programs have contributed to the local development of many positive public health efforts, including those aimed at pregnant women and children. Disease prevention, health promotion, screening, and health education have been particular foci.

Essentially, since the Great Society initiatives under President Lyndon Baines Johnson, the federal government has sought to restore and direct the overall public health effort in the United States. Directly, and indirectly in part as discussed in later sections of this chapter, the federal government, primarily through the Department of Health and Human Services, has provided fiscal support for public health and health services delivery as well as for substantial planning and strategy formulation efforts. Federal efforts to assess and define the nation's health and public health needs have resulted in the production of a number of seminal publications that essentially represent national health care goals. These are codified in such publications as the Institute of Medicine's report *Healthy People 2010*, which assesses the nation's status with regard to various health-related indicators and identifies national goals in various categories of measurable performance for both the public health system and health care delivery system. The Office of the Surgeon General in the Department of Health and Human Services as well as various parts of the Centers for Disease Control and Prevention, the Food and Drug Administration, the Office of Disease Prevention and Control, and other federal and quasi-federal agencies combined with staff and committees of the U. S. Congress all jointly are the de facto policy setting and strategic planning directorates for our nation's health care system to the extent that such efforts exist.

Government's Responsibility

Local public health agencies typically perform the duties listed in Table 5.1. These agencies are constantly monitoring and protecting the health of the population. Services range from assessing the cleanliness of restaurants and their compliance with health codes to protecting the water and food supplies of the community.

Public health agencies have a history dating back to the founding of the country. Indeed, the Plymouth Colony compiled vital statistics, such as births and deaths. One of the earliest boards of health in Boston in the late 1700s was headed by Paul Revere.

Local public health departments usually conduct ongoing disease surveillance and monitoring to determine if there are unusual outbreaks of infectious disease. They also assess disease patterns that may represent a threat to the community, such as AIDS. Local health departments are usually responsible for the frontline collection of vital sta-

tistics. Birth and death certificates are filed with the local health department, forwarded for statewide collection, and then moved onward for further compilation at the national level.

Local health departments have responsibility for a broad array of environmental health activities. These efforts are of immense importance to the welfare of the community, particularly in protecting the water, food, and milk supplies. Ongoing monitoring of these supplies and enforcement of local health codes are vital functions of health departments. Local health departments also usually conduct a variety of frontline health services including screening programs, health education, preventive efforts, such as immunization and vaccination programs, and

Table 5.1. Typical Services Provided by Local Health Departments

Vital statistics collection
Sanitation inspections
Health education
Cancer, hypertension, diabetes screening
Maintenance of disease registries
Epidemiology
Supervision of water and sewage systems
Monitoring biological attacks
Insect control
Environmental health
Dairy product supervision
Information services to physicians
Public health nursing services
Tuberculosis screening
Immunization/vaccination
Operation of health centers
Mental health centers
Family planning clinics
Venereal disease clinics
Terrorism preparedness
Emergency mobilization

operate clinics for specific diseases, such as venereal disease.

Since the September 11, 2001, terrorist attacks on the United States, local health departments have assumed a much more significant role in monitoring for potential biological threats and attacks. In addition, local public health departments have greatly enhanced their roles and responsibilities for community-wide preparations to respond to such a terrorist attack. Increased financial support, primarily from federal and state governments, has facilitated these efforts, but in most communities the complexity of the challenge and the availability of financial resources still leaves much to be desired. New technologies such as multiple monitoring stations, enhanced and more effective reporting networks, and much better organized response teams have enhanced our level of preparation. However, the potential threat from terrorist activity still remains a serious concern in most communities, particularly in major urban areas and in those cities perceived as potential targets. Terrorist monitoring and preparedness will for the foreseeable future be a new, ongoing, and expanded responsibility of local health departments throughout the nation.

Local health departments are further supported by state health departments. State responsibilities are listed in Table 5.2. When local health departments fail to adequately perform necessary and statutorily required functions, state departments usually have the authority to intervene and conduct those activities. State health departments are also responsible for setting statewide priorities, for compiling state vital statistics and other data, for the conduct of the state Medicaid program, for terrorism preparedness support, and for many other activities.

Federal support for public health services includes grants to local areas, compilation and analysis of national health-related and vital statistics data, support for state and local departments in clinical laboratory testing, particularly for more complex or obscure problems, and for ongoing disease surveillance.

Table 5.2. Typical Services Provided by State Public Health Departments

Personnel licensing boards
Hospital licensing
Nursing home licensing
Vital statistics collection
Health planning
Health data systems
Chronic disease surveillance
Communicable disease surveillance
State laboratory services
Development of immunization programs
Tuberculosis control
Veterinary public health
Administration of categorical programs
Emergency medical services
Terrorism preparedness
Support for direct health programs

The nature of public health departments and services, and their duties and obligations, have been a function of the political, economic, and social fabric of the country and have changed over time. As the role of government in health care has evolved, the duties of public health agencies have also changed.

PUBLIC HEALTH AND PREVENTION

The role of public health services in prevention is critical to the nation's health. The substantial decline in mortality in the United States in the twentieth century is primarily a function of public health and preventive services. Continuing surveillance and intervention are essential to ensure that the public's health is protected against the ravages of present and future disease threats. In addition, many of society's self-inflicted causes of morbidity and mortality, such as accidents, smoking, and work-site accidents, require intervention by public health officials.

Clinical preventive services are those specific services offered by physicians and other practitioners directly to patients on a one-to-one basis. Clinical preventive services include screening for various diseases including hypertension and various types of cancer. The appropriateness of the services and the frequency with which they are performed for otherwise healthy populations are the subject of various national studies and reports and are associated with a high level of controversy. Most clinical preventive services have a modest, but not insignificant, cost that must be weighed against the potential benefits on a population basis to assess the financial viability of performing such services.

The current biomedical revolution includes substantial efforts directed toward improving the specificity of various preventive screening methods. The results of these efforts will yield more cost-effective and accurate screening techniques, probably at lower costs. These efforts will substantially improve the detection and earlier treatment of many categories of disease, especially for cancer.

Preventive services that are provided to ensure the health of a population and to avert disease and illness are termed primary prevention. These efforts are the first line of protection for a population and are frequently the most effective in reducing illness and suffering and protecting against terrorism. Primary prevention, however, can be quite expensive, as is illustrated by the billions of dollars spent reducing air and water pollution over the years.

Specific clinical intervention provided to individual patients is secondary prevention. Secondary prevention is focused on preventing illness from progressing to a point where intervention is either highly complex or expensive. Screening individuals who have high disease risk based on previous medical or family history, or genetic indicators for specific diseases such as breast cancer, is an example of secondary prevention.

Tertiary prevention is focused on reducing the impact of diseases once they occur in individual patients. Thus, an individual who has already experienced a significant illness would be given medical guidance and recommendations to reduce further debilitating outcomes from such an illness.

Because it is difficult to measure the specific payoffs in many forms of prevention and in the application of clinical preventive services, there is a high degree of uncertainty and controversy regarding exactly when each of these measures should be offered and the extent to which they should be implemented for an entire population. The debate is highly significant given the costs involved in screening large numbers of people on a routine or periodic basis. In addition, virtually all screening involves the potential for both false-positive and false-negative results that can lead to either failure to follow-up with additional care when needed, or the provision of what eventually becomes unnecessary or inappropriate care.

Preventive services are integrally related to the overall quality of care provided to individuals and populations. Preventing the occurrence of disease is always better than treating disease once it occurs. The human toll associated with disease alone justifies considerable effort being directed toward prevention.

Ultimately, prevention is the principal goal. Unfortunately, the complexities of our society and of individual behavior make it much more difficult than might be expected to implement comprehensive preventive plans for populations. In addition, providers and insurers may lack the incentive to invest in preventive services, since most will not pay off for many years. The role of government and the trade-off between individual freedoms and society's interest in preventing disease are also serious considerations in weighing the extent to which preventive services should be implemented in a society.

Few people would argue against the prevention of illness and disease. But many complex and practical considerations enter into these deliberations. Combined with the many uncertainties involved in providing such services, the answers become much more difficult to discern for large populations such as ours.

THE ROLE OF THE FEDERAL GOVERNMENT IN PUBLIC HEALTH SERVICES

The federal government is actively involved in the design and provision of preventive services for the United States' population in many ways. A number of federal agencies are key to these efforts. These include the U. S. Department of Health and Human Services, which is the principal federal agency responsible for health related activities; the Veterans Administration, which has responsibility for providing health care services, including some preventive and public health services, to U. S. military veterans; and the various military services of the Department of Defense, which have responsibility for providing preventive and personal health services for active duty military persons and, in some instances, their dependents as well.

The federal Department of Homeland Security is the latest new agency to have a role related to public health services. In this instance, the department's role relates to the surveillance and preparation for a response to any biological, chemical, or related terrorist threat. In a broad sense, much of what the Department of Homeland Security does on a daily basis is public health. However, in a more traditional and narrow definition, only those components of the department's efforts related to population health and specifically to threats from biological and chemical agents would be most clearly classified in the realm of public health services.

The Department of Health and Human Services is an umbrella organization composed of a number of agencies with specific health-related responsibilities. The Department of Health and Human Services also includes a variety of agencies with responsibility for human services. However, human services, particularly in such areas as long-term care and mental health services, are integral to the public's health.

One of the most important agencies of the Department of Health and Human Services is the Centers for Disease Control and Prevention. This agency is responsible for monitoring the health status of the population and for conducting epidemiological investigations of disease outbreaks. This agency also provides support to state and local health departments throughout the nation. The agency's Epidemic Intelligence Service (EIS) sends out epidemiologists to investigate specific outbreaks of disease that could threaten communities anywhere in the United States.

The Department of Health and Human Services also includes the Food and Drug Administration (FDA). This agency is responsible for the approval of marketing for all ethical drugs and medical devices. Drugs and medical devices must be shown to be safe and efficacious before they are approved for use in the United States. This is an important function to ensure that the technological capabilities utilized in fighting illness are legitimate, and that they meet safety criteria.

The FDA is constantly weighing the costs and rigor of clinical review processes against economic concerns and the timeliness of the review process for new drugs and devices. Certain promising drugs for very serious diseases may even be given expedited review. In addition, the role of the FDA is largely defined by Congressional legislation. Political pressure has led Congress to exempt certain herbal and naturally occurring products from FDA approval such that the efficacy of these products does not need to be demonstrated through scientific approaches prior to their marketing to the general public. This controversial situation, in contrast to the rules and regulations promulgated for the ethical drug industry, is a clear example of political intervention in an otherwise generally scientifically directed review process.

The Centers for Medicare and Medicaid Services (CMS) is responsible for the federal role in the operation of the Medicare and Medicaid programs. This agency directly runs the Medicare program, although claims administration is conducted through fiscal intermediaries. The agency participates with each state in the administration, principally by the states, of the Medicaid program.

Another unit of the Department of Health and Human Services is the National Center for Health Statistics, responsible for the collection and analysis of health status and biostatistics data for the nation. Other units within the Department of Health and Human Services, including the National Institutes of Health and the Alcohol, Drug Abuse, and Mental Health Administration, either conduct internal or fund extramural biomedical research to advance our state of knowledge about illness and disease.

PREVENTIVE SERVICES AND HEALTH CARE PROVIDERS

Ultimately, preventing illness and disease is the responsibility of both providers and consumers. As noted previously in this book, individual consumers need to focus on their own behaviors as they pertain to their health and well-being. Individuals need to limit their participation in risky activities, work on improving their health and nutrition through exercise and diet, reduce levels of stress, and avoid accidents, workplace injuries, and the like.

As noted, government assumes a substantial burden in helping to ensure the health of the population. Of course, there are significant limits to the role that government can assume in a democratic society. In addition, there are significant cost trade-offs in the role of government. Resources and freedoms are always limited.

Frontline health care providers and insurers and other organizational entities involved in the delivery of health care services also assume a strategic role in ensuring the health of their patients. Increasingly, managed care organizations are assuming responsibility for more people; they also have enhanced responsibilities for prevention and health promotion. Patient education, screening services performed routinely on a periodic basis, and other direct interventions provide an opportunity for providers to enhance the patient's health and well-being. Patient compliance with provider

recommendations of course remains a significant barrier. In addition, many providers are reluctant to intervene too aggressively in their patients' personal lives.

Many managed care organizations, and even traditional insurance plans, have directed their attention toward determining which preventive services and patient education efforts pay off for both the populations they serve and their own bottom lines. Although our nation appears to be at a transition point, ultimately it will be in the best interest of all concerned to accurately determine where preventive interventions can benefit both patients and payers. Managed care organizations and insurers ultimately have tremendous leverage to influence patient and provider behavior in the provision of preventive and health promotion services. The use of this leverage, performed in a politically acceptable manner, will have tremendous long-term pay offs for our nation.

THE ULTIMATE PUBLIC HEALTH SYSTEM

Eventually, and ideally, our nation needs to meld together all of these perspectives and opportunities for prevention in the areas of health promotion and public health. All parties must participate in ensuring the nation's health with a tremendous focused effort on preventing illness and disease rather than just treating it after it occurs. Since the ultimate goal of a health care system is the reduction of morbidity and mortality, improvement of functional status, and the reduction of pain and suffering, it would seem that all parties have consistent objectives in this area. The role of government, especially in such matters as mandated benefits and hospital stays, needs to be further addressed.

The economic and political advantages, combined with the eventual ability of technology to improve the tools utilized for preventive services, will lead to greater enhancement of the public's health. In the interim, greater delineation of responsibility for improving health on the part of patients, providers, insurers, and employers is essential. Emphasis on biomedical research that will lead to better techniques for the prevention and detection of disease must also be a high priority for the nation. Enhanced delivery of technology, access to mammography, disease and pregnancy testing, and protection of privacy, is essential. We can all concur that avoiding disease is better than treating it and that the application of a myriad of approaches for such avoidance should be a high national priority.

Employers also play a key role in public health and preventive services. In particular, employers hold a special responsibility to ensure the safety of their workers through occupational health efforts. The sometimes controversial involvement of the federal Occupational and Safety Health Administration (OSHA) and its state counterparts has led to substantial reductions in workplace morbidity and mortality. Although these regulatory efforts have often met with political opposition, many employers recognize the value of a safe work environment. Employers today also struggle with many newly recognized challenges, such as employees with disabilities, the unique problems associated with computer use, various ergonomic concerns, and vehicular accidents in the work environment. In addition, as payers for health care services, employers also have a key role in promoting health and safety through the delivery of health care services to employees and their families. Finally, employers have tremendous political leverage to promote health and safety issues in each community level and to formulate national policy to promote the public's health throughout the nation.

STUDY QUESTIONS

1. What are public health and clinical preventive services?
2. What is the role of the federal government in prevention and public health?
3. What are the roles of state and local health departments in protecting the nation's health?
4. What are the levels of prevention services?
5. What trade-offs in costs, personal rights, and freedom are inherent in public health issues?
6. What role should employers and insurers play in prevention?
7. Describe the major economic, social, political, and technological forces that shaped the development of public health services in the United States over the past 100 years.
8. Who makes public health policy and how is such policy established and promulgated?

CHAPTER 6

Hospitals and Health Systems

Chapter Objectives

1. To describe the history and evolution of the nation's hospitals.
2. To explain how the nation's hospitals are utilized by our citizens.
3. To describe different avenues for hospital ownership.
4. To outline the development of hospital and health systems.
5. To address the challenges that face the nation's hospital system.

The nature of the American hospital has changed dramatically since its inception as an almshouse in the 1800s. Originally created to care for the poor during sickness, while the middle and upper classes were cared for at home, the hospital has evolved into the repository of our nation's most technologically advanced health care resources.

Recently, the hospital's role has become more complex, buffeted by numerous economic, social, political, and technological forces. In addition, the role of the hospital in our society and its future viability have become inextricably interwoven with the financial mechanisms created to pay for health care services.

The hospital industry has also become increasingly embroiled in controversy associated with issues of governance, reimbursement, malpractice liability, and relationships with physicians and other organizations. Aggressive government enforcement of various rules and regulations associated with the Medicare program have led to serious legal action against individuals and organizations in the industry. At the same time, increasing pressure for public accountability, and enhancement of the quality of care, combined with a range of pressures from hospital medical staff, physicians, and patients, have further complicated the world of hospital administration.

This chapter relates the evolving role of the hospital in the health care industry, describes its structure and organization, and reveals its current challenges and future directions. The changing nature of the hospital dramatically reflects changes in the way our nation's health care system is structured and financed.

HISTORY OF THE AMERICAN HOSPITAL

The hospital, even in its current form, reflects its traditions of service and caring. Born out of society's need to provide a place to care for those both ill and poor in our society, the hospital has a well-established tradition of service and charity. While today's hospital is run in a much more businesslike manner than in the past, the commitment to the community and to patients remains exceedingly strong. However, these commitments are constantly challenged by the stresses associated with the financing of health care services.

As medical technology has evolved and as medicine has become increasingly specialized, the hospital has assumed a more important role in medical education. In the early 1900s, medical education was poorly organized and not particularly scientifically based.

In 1910, Abraham Flexner examined the nation's medical schools and wrote a scathing report that resulted in an extensive reorganization of medical education. As a result of the Flexner report, medical education became much more rigorous, more hospital oriented, and more scientific. Many medical schools closed, as well.

In this new environment, the hospital assumed an increasingly important role as the institutional base for medical education. With greater specialization after World War II, and a heavy dependence on technology, medical education became largely based in teaching hospitals. Over the last 25 years, the increasing use of noninstitutional settings has shifted some aspects of medical education from the inpatient to outpatient sectors, but the hospital continues to play the key role in health professions education.

As for physicians, nursing education also evolved largely around the hospital. The era of modern nursing, which has included the work of such luminaries as Florence Nightingale, has seen growing professionalism in the nursing field. The hospital has become a significant institutional focus for the technically complex roles of nursing. Since World War II, specialization and technology have required greater technical training for hospital-based nurses.

The duties of many other health care professionals have been created or expanded with the hospital-based technological advances of the twentieth century. Thus, the hospital sector has played a key role in the training and employment of professionals in many health care fields.

The nation's hospitals are a diverse group of organizations with many different historical and evolutionary backgrounds. Although some of the nation's hospitals began as facilities to care for the poor with little access to medical services, others rapidly developed into teaching institutions for the developing scientifically based medical schools. From their early origins, many hospitals affiliated with each other through various religious or charitable entities. Others were started by physicians or by other for-profit companies and some were created by government entities or by corporate parents. Hospitals have had to respond dramatically over the years to changes in the practice of medicine including new technologies, the expansion of surgical and diagnostic procedures, the vast proliferation of imaging technologies, and changes in the organization and delivery of health care. Community needs, charitable donor preferences, physician demands, and patient perceptions have all radically affected the design, development, and operation of the nation's hospitals. Governmental funding, particularly through the Medicare and Medicaid programs, also radically altered the evolution of hospitals as they responded to the parameters for reimbursement established by these programs. Similarly, managed care and its approach to negotiating contractual arrangements with hospitals has also had a dramatic impact on how hospitals function.

In recent years, the central role of inpatient services in the hospital has continued to expand with a focus on increasingly specialized services. However, the hospital as an institution has broadened its role and, in advanced environments, serves as the focal point for organizing the broad spectrum of health care services.

Increasing integration of health care systems and the need to provide comprehensive services for purposes of contracting with employers and insurers, particularly under managed care, have forced hospitals into many other related businesses, such as ambulatory care and home health services. At the same time, an increasing shift of services from inpatient to outpatient settings, and the need to retain referral business for inpatient and specialty services, have also broadened the scope of hospital care.

At the present time, as an example of recent industry changes, perhaps 70 percent of all surgical services are performed on an ambulatory basis without overnight hospitalization. Hospitals that ignore such trends are in jeopardy of becoming isolated islands of tertiary services with limited revenue sources and without enough referrals to assure an ample supply of patients for inpatient services.

The industry has also seen changes in the roles of for-profit hospitals and health systems, increasing both vertical and horizontal integration, consolidation and specialization, and increasing competition from a variety of sources. The hospital industry as a large institutional provider of expensive services has been targeted in a variety of ways by government reimbursement policy and politicians as well as by private voluntary health insurance companies and other managed care organizations. Increasing standards for accreditation, specialty certification, licensure, and for participation in a variety of public and private programs have also occurred over the past 20 years. Patient expectations, in part the result of enhanced biomedical knowledge and mass media attention to clinical issues, has also increased while at the same time exposure of financial, clinical, and access flaws in the industry by the media, government, and private watchdog organizations has alerted the public to the need for further improvement in how the industry provides care and the control over services.

The evolution of the hospital as an institution has challenged the industry to shift from its historical, limited perspectives and devotion to inpatient care into a much broader perspective covering a wide array of inpatient and ambulatory services. Coupled with these trends is the concurrent evolution of technology, dramatic changes in the financing of institutional services, and the growing pressures for cost containment and quality assurance arising from managed care. Today's hospital is truly challenged to live in a world different from its comfortable, historical origins.

CHARACTERISTICS OF AMERICAN HOSPITALS

There are approximately 5,000 non-federal, short-term, acute-care hospitals in the United States. Long-term facilities for individuals with chronic illness and various specialty hospitals exist as well. Table 6.1 indicates the distribution of these hospitals by ownership category.

Since hospitals grew out of a charity mission, it is not surprising that the majority of hospitals are not-for-profit entities. Ownership as a not-for-profit hospital, generally under Section 501c3 of the U.S. Internal Revenue Code, signifies an entity that is owned and operated for the public welfare and for which there is no equity or stock ownership.

Table 6.1 also indicates the distribution of the nation's short-stay hospitals by hospital size. The majority of the nation's hospitals have fewer than 200 licensed beds. The largest hospitals tend to be teaching facilities and tertiary care medical centers. Many small and rural hospitals have 50 or fewer beds. These hospitals have difficulty operating efficiently and maintaining financial viability owing to the necessity for maintaining a range of basic services and facilities, almost always with limited overall demand.

There is a greater predominance of larger facilities in the East, with fewer such hospitals in the western part of the country. This is the result of a trend toward the construction of smaller (100- to 350-bed) hospitals in more recent years, concurrent with the movement of population westward.

Table 6.1 indicates that there are approximately 1 million hospital beds currently in the United States. Hospital occupancy rates by ownership and size of hospital also provide evidence of inefficiency, since the average hospital in the country operates at only about 66 percent overall occupancy. Teaching

hospitals and tertiary care medical centers tend to have higher occupancy rates, and small hospitals tend to have especially low occupancy.

There is tremendous variability in hospital utilization across the nation and even in individual communities. Changes in population density as a result of immigration and movement of population with geographic boundaries can dramatically change the market for hospital services even in an individual community. Since hospitals are large, expensive structures built to withstand many years of use, their capabilities and facilities can quickly become outmoded as technology changes. In addition, populations served can change in characteristics and location. Finally, the increasing predominance of managed care and associated contracting mechanisms can dramatically change a hospital's market and geographic service area over a relatively short time frame.

Tables 6.2 and 6.3 present information on the use of the nation's hospitals. Overall, hospital length of stay averages 4.9 days, with 115 discharges per 1,000 people per year. Hospital use increases significantly with age, is greater for blacks and the poor, and is notably higher in the South and the Northeast.

The relationship between hospital efficiency, size, and occupancy is extremely important in achieving national cost containment objectives. The optimal size for a hospital is probably between 150 and 250 beds, and the ideal occupancy rate is likely around 85 percent. Hospitals should be large enough to achieve efficiencies of scale but not so large as to become highly bureaucratic. Hospital occupancy should be high enough to achieve maximum efficiencies but not so high as to be unable to meet the peaks in demand that occur from time to time.

In recent years, the emergence of new biological threats such as the severe acute respiratory syndrome (SARS) epidemic and recognition of continuing threats from influenza and other long-standing infectious diseases has combined with the need to be prepared to respond to possible terrorist attacks that involve mass injuries or deaths. These challenges continually face the hospital industry partic-

Table 6.1. Short-Stay Hospitals, Beds, and Occupancy Rates, According to Type of Ownership and Size of Hospital: United States, 1975 and 2001

Type of Ownership and Size of Hospital	1975	2001	Type of Ownership and Size of Hospital	1975	2001
	Number			Percentage of beds occupied	
Hospitals			**Occupancy rate**		
All hospitals	7,156	5,801	All hospitals	76.7	66.7
Federal	382	243	Federal	80.7	69.8
Nonfederal	6,774	5,558	Nonfederal	76.3	66.5
Community	5,875	4,908	Community	75.0	64.5
Nonprofit	3,339	2,998	Nonprofit	77.5	65.8
Proprietary	775	754	Proprietary	65.9	57.0
State-local government	1,761	1,156	State-local government	70.4	64.1
6–99 beds	2,935	2,267	6–99 beds	56.5	49.2
100–199 beds	1,363	1,289	100–199 beds	71.2	60.7
200–299 beds	678	635	200–299 beds	77.1	65.5
300–399 beds	378	348	300–399 beds	79.7	66.4
400–499 beds	230	191	400–499 beds	81.1	68.9
500 beds or more	291	249	500 beds or more	80.9	72.8
Beds					
All hospitals	1,465,828	987,440			
Federal	131,946	51,900			
Nonfederal	1,333,882	935,540			
Community	941,844	825,966			
Nonprofit	658,195	585,070			
Proprietary	73,495	108,718			
State-local government	210,154	132,178			
6–99 beds	154,174	115,151			
100–199 beds	192,438	174,024			
200–299 beds	164,405	154,420			
300–399 beds	127,728	119,753			
400–499 beds	101,278	84,745			
500 beds or more	201,821	177,873			

ularly in urban areas and have raised serious questions about the ideal occupancy rates for hospitals such that adequate emergency capacity could be available in the event of a significant community challenge.

Hospital Ownership

Not-for-profit hospitals are typically community-based facilities but also include university teaching hospitals and other organizations. Not-for-profit hospitals raise

Table 6.2. Discharges, Days of Care, and Average Length of Stay in Nonfederal Hospitals, Selected Characteristics: United States, Selected Years

Characteristic	Discharges per 1,000 Population		Days of Care per 1,000 Population		Average Length of Stay in Days	
	1980	2001*	1980	2001*	1980	2001*
Total	173.4	115.3	1,297.0	563.2	7.5	4.9
Age						
Under 18 years	75.6	43.4	341.4	192.7	4.5	4.4
18–44 years	155.3	87.6	818.6	323.6	5.3	3.7
45–54 years	174.8	94.5	1,314.9	455.9	7.5	4.8
55–64 years	215.4	139.3	1,889.4	732.4	8.8	5.3
65 years and older	383.7	354.9	4,098.3	2,067.8	10.7	5.8
Sex						
Male	153.2	100.2	1,239.7	535.7	8.1	5.3
Female	195.0	130.9	1,365.2	592.9	7.0	4.5
Geographic region						
Northeast	162.0	129.0	1,400.6	733.6	8.6	5.7
Midwest	192.1	115.6	1,484.8	532.6	7.7	4.6
South	179.7	124.7	1,262.3	622.1	7.0	5.0
West	150.5	98.5	956.9	461.4	6.4	4.7

*1999 for geographic region data.

capital by borrowing in the bond market and through donations from philanthropy. Historically, philanthropic contributions were a major source of capital for hospital development and operations, particularly for those hospitals serving the poor. Philanthropy now accounts for a very small percentage of the capital, and particularly operating expense, budgets of not-for-profit hospitals.

Not-for-profit hospitals can earn a profit, although it is not called that. Any excess of revenue over expenses in a not-for-profit hospital is utilized for the further development of the hospital and its services. In certain circumstances, as discussed further later, a not-for-profit hospital can be operated by a for-profit corporation, so that ownership should be considered separately from the operating entity.

A second category of hospital ownership is the for-profit corporation. For-profit hospitals had their origins in facilities developed, owned, and operated by physicians. It is rare today for a hospital to be owned by its physicians, although this was much more common many years ago. The potential for conflicts of interest is obvious in such an arrangement. To protect against such conflicts there is now a variety of federal and state laws regulating physician ownership of those facilities, such as clinical laboratories to which they refer their patients.

Today's for-profit hospital is typically owned by a national hospital company. Fewer hospitals are now independently owned on a for-profit basis as solo, free-standing institutions than in past years.

For-profit hospitals and systems can raise capital through the equity markets, and these corporations are owned through the issuance of stock. Publicly held, for-profit companies trade on the New York and other stock exchanges, and an equity investment in

Table 6.3. Discharges, Days of Care, and Average Length of Stay in Nonfederal Hospitals by Race, Poverty Status, and Insurance: United States, 2001

Characteristic	Discharges per 1,000 population	Days of Care per 1,000 population	Average Length of Stay in Days
Total	122.0	554.2	4.5
Race			
White only	93.2	369.4	4.0
Black or African American only	130.3	657.2	5.0
American Indian and Alaska Native only	169.2	767.6	4.5
Asian only	68.0	228.7	3.4
Poverty status			
Poor	167.9	857.7	5.1
Near poor	136.2	646.5	4.7
Nonpoor	86.5	316.7	3.7
Health insurance status			
Insured	104.3	433.2	4.2
Private	84.4	311.8	3.7
Medicaid	296.2	1,495.1	5.0
Uninsured	64.2	270.9	4.2

these entities is available to anyone who purchases their stock. Other for-profit hospitals and systems are privately held; their stock is not publicly available.

For-profit entities can raise capital through the issuance of debt and through the reinvestment of profits (retained earnings). Unlike not-for-profit hospitals, which do not pay any income taxes and are often exempt from local real estate taxes, for-profit entities pay the full range of federal, state, and local taxes.

For-profit companies often manage hospitals under contract to other owners. For example, as mentioned previously, a hospital can be owned by a nonprofit entity but be managed under contract by a for-profit hospital management company.

Hospital management companies use their expertise to own and operate their own hospitals and to sell their management skills to other owners.

Another category of hospital ownership is the government hospital, owned by the federal, state, or local government. At the federal level, this category includes the 163 hospitals that are part of the Veterans Administration system and the military hospitals that are located throughout the nation and the world. State hospitals include, most notably, state mental health, long-term care, and local short-term, acute-care hospitals, including county hospitals and those owned by other jurisdictions, such as hospital districts. Governmentally owned hospitals can also be managed by for-profit or not-for-profit companies under contractual arrangements.

Regardless of ownership, most hospitals throughout the nation require similar management, financial support, technology, and other resources. Hospitals may differ in ways of raising capital, the payment of taxes, specific goals and missions, marketing functions, the nature of clientele, and contracts for care. In addition, governmental hospitals typically operate under a politically allocated annual budget.

All hospitals require the use of modern management techniques, including computer-based information systems, to function in today's competitive environment. There is considerable controversy as to whether for-profit management companies and hospitals are more efficient and the extent to which the quality of care provided is comparable in for-profit and not-for-profit settings.

Among the arguments frequently heard about the proprietary sector is that for-profit hospitals tend to ìskim the creamî by locating in areas where the local population has high levels of insurance coverage and good incomes. Such hospitals also allegedly shun highly specialized but lower-profit services, such as burn units.

Since these organizations are run for a profit and must provide a return on equity capital to their owners, it would seem prudent for them to provide services that are profitable. Such a philosophy would be consistent with our national economic system, leaving the uninsured and unprofitable services to governmental hospitals, which are the providers of last resort.

Another argument utilized in assessing the role of profit versus not-for-profit hospitals is that for-profit institutions, because of their profit motivation, are less likely to provide adequate levels of nursing care and other resources to the patient. There is mixed evidence with regard to these resource-based issues. On the one hand, we are using competitive markets to push hospitals to operate more efficiently; on the other hand, we also want them to maintain a high quality of care. These may be conflicting objectives.

There are probably many instances of both for-profit and not-for-profit hospitals limiting resource availability in patient care. Who does this best while maintaining the highest quality care is extremely difficult to determine. Some argue that the profit motive should not be a part of the health care industry. Nevertheless, physicians and most other providers have, since the origins of the nation's health care system, operated on a for-profit basis.

HOSPITAL ORGANIZATION AND MANAGEMENT

Hospitals typically have three sources of power and authority in their organizational structure. The first, the hospital board of trustees or directors, is ultimately responsible for the operation of the facility. The composition of the board will vary from hospital to hospital. The board is generally composed of knowledgeable individuals, often with health care expertise. The board's role is to direct the overall operation of the hospital and to delegate specific duties to the hospital's administration and medical staff.

Hospital administration, the second source of power and authority, is responsible for the day-to-day operation of the facility. The hospital administrator or chief executive officer (CEO) is the key individual in the management structure. Various assistant and associate administrators report to the CEO. Department heads and other operating personnel, in turn, report to these managers. Multihospital systems may have more complex administrative structures with individual facility administrators reporting to corporate managers at the regional or national levels.

The medical staff is the third source of power and authority in the hospital. The medical staff derives its authority from the delegation of responsibility on the part of the hospital's board. The medical staff is organized according to its by-laws, usually with elected officers. The medical staff represents the physicians, usually community-based, who provide care within the hospital. In today's complex environment some, or even all, of the hospital's physicians may be under contract to the hospital. In addition, hospitals are increasingly aligning their interests with those of the medical staffs through joint ventures, contractual arrangements for services, and the development of physician hospital organizations (PHOs).

The medical staff is usually headed by the medical director, chief of staff, or the president of the medical staff. Hospital administration may employ a physician-manager to deal with medical issues; this person often has the title of vice president of medical affairs. Hospitals increasingly employ physicians in a variety of full- and part-time positions delivering, supervising, or evaluating care. Some are clinical department heads with line authority.

The medical staff is responsible for the granting of privileges to physicians who work in the hospital and for admitting patients. Privileges are usually limited to a physician's areas of specialization. The more complex the hospital, the more specialized the medical staff. Often, the medical staff is further organized into specific clinical departments, such as for obstetrics and gynecology or pediatrics. The medical staff is also responsible for monitoring and ensuring the quality of care provided by its members. This function is carried out through various committees and the quality assurance staff.

Conflicts between these three sources of power and authority in the hospital are common. The medical staff, representing its physicians, often argues for the hospital's obtaining the latest in facilities and equipment. Administration is concerned about cost containment and competitive market pricing of services. The board must always look out for the hospital's overall financial viability, as well as its prestige, quality of care, growth, and long-term mission. In some hospitals, most notably those of the U.S. military, the interests of all three parties are closely aligned. Increasing vertical integration, contracting, and managed care are also forcing greater alliances among the parties in the hospital's organization.

In recent years, the hospital medical staff has faced increased pressures to address issues of efficiency, managed care contracting, and other less traditional concerns. Ultimately, hospitals must control the behavior of their physicians whether it be through the medical staff or through other mechanisms to better align physician interests with those of the institution. These issues are particularly important under managed care programs where risk has been shifted, through capitation and other mechanisms, to the provider.

In addition to greater control over physician clinical practice, other issues such as physician education, quality of care, compliance with medical regimens and clinical guidelines, and adherence to various administrative and governmental rules and regulations are also important concerns impinging on the relationship between institutions and their providers. The future role of the hospital medical staff and its relationship to these many complex issues of physician behavior will require further examination as the health care system continues to evolve in the future.

ISSUES OF CONCERN TO THE FUTURE OF THE AMERICAN HOSPITAL

Numerous trends and issues affect the nation's hospitals today. Some of the most important of these are discussed in this section. The continuing changes in

the health care industry mean that the hospital's role is never static, and the challenges faced by hospitals and their boards, administrators, and medical staffs continue to grow.

The Role of Technology

The hospital evolved from a place for the poor to the repository of the nation's technological prowess. This evolution has continued with the hospital increasingly being a source of more and more sophisticated inpatient services.

As more services are provided on an outpatient basis, the inpatient side of the hospital has increasingly offered care that requires an extremely high level of sophistication using complex technology. This "intensity of care" has contributed significantly to increasing costs for inpatient hospital services. Further, hospitals require more and more sophisticated employees to provide this increasingly complex care.

The use of fiberoptic surgical equipment now allows many patients to have procedures performed on an outpatient basis or to need only a minimal inpatient stay. For many patients, this substitutes a very short hospital stay for what was previously a 4- to 5-day hospitalization. However, such care is often expensive even with reduced costs for inpatient care.

Long-term substitution of noninvasive drug-based therapies for certain current surgical procedures could have a further dramatic impact on the nation's hospital system. Imaging has also seen a great explosion in both use and outpatient settings for services. Magnetic resonance and other more advanced technologies greatly facilitate both diagnosis and outpatient provision of services.

Technology will continue to be a driving factor in hospital costs and in the organization of services. Changing technology could substantially alter the hospital as we know it today. Nonsurgical therapies, for example, could eliminate the need for coronary artery bypass surgery. Technological change in the past has had dramatic effects on hospitals, as exemplified by the shift of approximately 70 percent of all surgery to the outpatient side.

Rural Hospitals

Rural hospitals, as indicated previously, generally experience low levels of bed occupancy. These hospitals face difficult financial and social pressures. They are expected to be readily available for routine care yet cannot realistically be held to the same standards of financial performance and efficiency as larger, urban hospitals.

Rural hospitals are prominent organizations in their communities. They are expected to fulfill a broader social mission than their urban counterparts. From a strictly financial point of view, closure of rural hospitals may make sense in many communities. However, the need to provide access to at least a minimum level of hospital care for a geographically disseminated population, community pride, and pragmatic issues of rapid response to local emergencies may mandate that we consider rural hospitals a unique resource.

Our society needs to determine reasonable travel expectations for people to obtain hospital care, such as labor and delivery, emergency treatment, and routine hospitalization. The role of the rural hospital and its staff needs to be carefully defined. Appropriate mechanisms must be built into the financial structure of the health care industry to permit these hospitals to function at a level sufficient to meet local community needs. Under President George W. Bush, efforts to do so have been pursued by enhancing reimbursements under Medicare.

Academic Medical Centers

Academic medical centers are the principal applied educational institutions for undergraduate (MD or DO) and postgraduate (internships, residencies, and fellowships) medical education. These institutions are often associated with universities and are located mostly in large urban communities. They face numerous challenges including the provision of care to medically underserved communities and to individuals needing the most complex and sophisticated technology. These centers are often responsible for a significant portion of our national biomedical research effort, particularly for applied clinical research.

Academic medical centers provide a full range of medical care services but are also viewed as a significant resource for the most sophisticated levels of care and as a referral base for other practitioners in the community. Much of the care provided in these institutions is a result of the medical education process, with patients being seen by medical students, residents, and faculty members of the medical schools with which they are associated. Because of the medical and research missions of these institutions, they differ significantly from traditional community hospitals in many respects including management approaches and costs.

Academic medical centers typically are not the most cost effective providers of health care. Teaching and research are expected activities that tend to be associated with higher costs of care. At the same time, the teaching and research missions of these institutions is fundamental to the future success of our medical care establishment. Of course no payer, government or private, wants to assume additional costs. However, someone somewhere has to pay for the costs of research and education in these institutions, and typically costs are somewhat increased for patients with the ability to pay themselves or through private insurance to help offset lower reimbursement from some government programs and for patients who have no financial resources. Cutbacks in the Medicare program in particular adversely affect academic medical centers because of their reliance on this source of funding. Increased penetration of managed care plans places further competitive pressures on pricing policies in academic medical centers. It is essential to the future of our nation's health that compensation arrangements are agreed on such that academic medical centers can

maintain their leadership in research and education while still being competitive in the health
care marketplace.

HOSPITAL EVOLUTION INTO HEALTH SYSTEMS

Increasing competition, and the pressures of cost
containment and managed care, have combined with
other factors to lead hospitals and other health care
organizations into a variety of alliances and other
forms of consolidation. Vertical integration, in which
the entire array of health care delivery organizations
are combined to form a comprehensive health care
delivery system, has become more popular.

Various forms of consolidation have left few
hospitals operating independently. The need to
provide insurers and employers with comprehensive, rather than fragmented, services, combined
with the economic advantages of being part of a
much larger organization, has resulted in mergers,
acquisitions, and other alliances. In addition, technological changes and the shift of services to the
ambulatory care arena have substantially changed
the nature of traditional hospital inpatient services.

Hospital consolidation often incorporates the
entire range of health care services into an organized delivery system through vertical integration.
Affiliation, or other arrangements among hospitals
themselves, such as cooperative purchasing organizations or multihospital companies, is typically
referred to as horizontal integration. Both of these
types of integration have become common in the
hospital industry over the past 25 years.

Financial pressures affecting hospital services
and organizations including the need for greater
efficiencies, an increasingly competitive marketplace, the need to reduce excess capacity, and the
need to eliminate redundancies and inefficiencies
have fueled these trends. The growth of for-profit
and not-for-profit multihospital systems has also
accelerated the trend toward consolidation.
Consolidation and horizontal and vertical integra-

tion can improve competitive positions in the marketplace, increase economic efficiencies, provide a
broader platform with which to negotiate contracts
under managed care with insurers and employers,
and provide better market coverage and control in
larger geographic areas.

Through vertical integration hospitals can affiliate
with other providers such as physician practices and
home health agencies to provide a broad spectrum
of health care services. The advantages of purchasing
from one vendor the full range of health care for
enrolled populations are many. This approach is also
attractive when used to shift costs and risk to the
provider organizations. In addition, there are potential efficiencies in contracting for a full range of services from one organization, which then assumes
responsibility for patient access to care, continuity of
services, and for the quality of care provided. In
addition, many forms of managed care represent the
ultimate in vertical integration by incorporating the
full range of services, and by providing the managerial and operational mechanisms for coordinating,
integrating, and evaluating the care that is provided.

Vertical integration can promote more appropriate use of resources since the delivery organization
controls the full range of health care settings.
Integrated information systems, which are becoming increasingly sophisticated, also serve to facilitate
the use of the most appropriate resources and the
overall management of these integrated networks.

Consolidation through vertical and horizontal
integration raises many complex issues. These
include, but are not limited to, concerns over
antitrust and market control as these systems
become larger and more powerful. Limitations on
patient access to care as a result of cost-containment
strategies may also impinge on the overall quality of
care provided. In the for-profit arena, questions
have been raised about the impact of the profit
motive on commitment to community needs and
on access and cost containment.

Horizontal and vertical integration in the hospital industry tends to be a dynamic process over
long periods of time. Some attempts at vertical

integration were not particularly successful, and in recent years some of hospital industry leaders have refocused their efforts on horizontal integration, relying on contractual arrangements for other services and for financing. Neither vertical nor horizontal integration is a guaranteed road to financial or operational success and both are highly complex arrangements and challenging in their execution.

Although vertical and horizontal integration has tremendous advantages and efficiencies when successful, considerable effort is required to achieve that success. Independently operating but linked organizations must have common goals and objectives, and resources must be utilized efficiently and in a manner that promotes such efficiency. Employees must also be on board and financial and nonfinancial incentives must align with organizational goals as well. Integration can potentially lead to greater cost effectiveness, better utilization controls, and other economies of scale. Management of integrated organizations must have the appropriate ability and authority to establish needed incentives and to monitor how well the organizations function. Vertical and horizontal integration of the health care system is inevitable, and a positive development, but one fraught with complex managerial challenges and the need for constant monitoring.

Ultimately, hospitals are responding to the highly complex environment in which they operate. They are also responding to the political, economic, and social forces that they have faced over the years. Trends in medical technology have substantially altered the nature of the hospital industry and its role in the marketplace. Such change is inevitable and desirable. We must continue to assure that needed services are provided in a manner that encourages the provision of high quality hospital care for all Americans.

For-Profit Hospitals and Health Systems

The complex issues regarding the role of for-profit hospitals and their function in the marketplace continue to elicit considerable debate. Recent evidence suggests that not-for-profit hospitals provide slightly more charity care than for-profit hospitals and are more likely to provide care to Medicaid patients. Not-for-profit hospitals have a greater tendency to be involved in medical education and biomedical research and to provide more complex tertiary care such as burn services or organ transplantation. The quality of care provided in for-profit hospitals is probably as good as if not better than that provided in the not-for-profit sector, although many such measures are difficult to assess.

Whether for-profit hospitals are more efficient is an extremely complex question, and recent evidence suggests that they may not be. For-profit hospitals may be more likely to earn their profits by better managing the services they offer and the locations in which they operate.

THE FUTURE OF THE AMERICAN HOSPITAL

The hospital has evolved dramatically over time. It is a dynamic organization that responds to many influences in its environment. These include the technology of modern medicine and how that technology is delivered to patients, as well as numerous economic, social, political, and environmental factors.

Hospitals are always in the firing line and today face many difficult challenges. In many areas of the country, hospitals have encountered significant shortages of nursing personnel. Pay and working conditions, among other factors, have led hospitals to rely on hourly contract nurses and to face a difficult recruitment environment. States that mandate nurse to patient ratios have put further pressure on nursing recruitment and retention in their hospitals. For their part, nurses tend to be overworked and sometimes underpaid and, at the least, are at the forefront of dealing with increasingly demanding patients who seek excellence and the availability of the best technology. Hospitals, at the same time, are also under fire for deaths attributable to medical errors (see references in the Appendix). Patient safety is an increasingly important issue and is focusing concern on the accuracy of medical records, drug interactions, and numerous other concerns. Patient privacy is another major new area of concern as a result of recent federal legislation that in fact further complicates the care process. Changes in federal Medicare and Medicaid program provisions further complicate the lives of hospital managers. The Balanced Budget Act of 1997 and recent changes in the laws pertaining to Medicare have established many new requirements, provisions, and programs and a variety of demonstrations to test additional changes that might be recommended in the future. Finally, managed care programs and providers have increasingly demanded more substantial discounts in contractual reimbursement arrangements as well as a variety of reporting and quality assurance mechanisms.

In recent years, the hospital has been dramatically altered by the forces of managed care, insurance contracting, technology, governmental regulation, and institutional reimbursement. The dramatic shift of services from the inpatient to the outpatient sectors has altered the mix and intensity of care provided in the hospital. These trends are likely to continue in the future.

STUDY QUESTIONS

1. How did the nation's hospital system evolve during the twentieth century?
2. What are the ownership characteristics of the nation's hospitals?
3. How often and by whom are the nation's hospitals used?
4. What are the differences between for-profit and not-for-profit hospitals?
5. To what extent are multihospital systems changing the nature of the hospital industry?
6. What are the problems faced by small rural hospitals?
7. How is the hospital likely to evolve in the future, particularly considering changes in technology, financing, and the organization of delivery systems?

CHAPTER 7

Mental and Behavioral Health Services

Chapter Objectives

1. To describe the history of mental health services in the United States.
2. To contrast the differences between private and public mental health services.
3. To discuss the use of inpatient mental health facilities.
4. To explain the role of different health care personnel in the mental health field.
5. To state how mental health services are paid for.
6. To examine the future of mental health services in the United States.

Mental and behavioral health services and long-term care services, the subject of the next chapter, are areas in the nation's health care system that are poised for fundamental change and dramatic growth. Mental health services, in particular, increasingly involve the use of the medical model for solutions to patient problems.

While traditional definitions of mental illness center around the manifestations of alterations in thinking and behavior that cause inappropriate or nonconforming attitudes, interactions, and activity, the increasing role of somatic etiology or causes is leading to a reassessment of mental health. This change in attitude and approach is empowering changes in societal attitudes, health care delivery, and financing for mental health-related conditions. Mental health needs cross all strata of our society and are exceedingly common throughout an individual's lifetime. Although a relatively smaller proportion of all citizens, perhaps 3 percent, suffer from more severe forms of mental illness, the common expressions of mental health needs are seen in many more people each year, including the very young and the very old.

Many manifestations of mental illness also result from the increasing dissolution of traditional family structures and the increasing stress in living in a very complex and often challenging world. Poverty, workplace stresses, family and social pressures, and many other influences exacerbate each individual's efforts to reach a satisfactory level of functioning within our society. Many of our society's social and economic problems, such as domestic and workplace violence, hazardous driving habits, child abuse, family instability, problems related to sexual activity, homelessness, and unemployment also contribute greatly to these problems. Mental health needs are vast and are at least partially based in larger societal issues, presenting immense challenges that face our health care system in addressing mental health needs for all Americans.

The dramatic results of biomedical research in recent years have increased the number of mental health diagnoses for which drug therapies are now available. Work in progress, and especially drugs in the research pipeline, will greatly expand the armament of psychotropic drugs available for treating an ever-wider array of mental health problems. At the same time, some traditional, nondrug-based therapies, a few of which have been called into question, have continued to be widely utilized for certain types of patient needs.

The increasing thrust of mental health therapies is to apply the medical model, primarily using psychotropic drugs. This will mainstream mental health services and alleviate many of the past concerns of insurers. The history of mental health services in the United States reflects a past different from what may be anticipated for the future.

HISTORICAL PRECEDENTS IN MENTAL HEALTH

Modern mental health services have a recent history. Conversely, mental illness has a long, despicable record of inadequate attention in the United States. Unlike somatic illness and public health services, which have a relatively distinguished track record dating back to the founding of our nation, the mental health field has long struggled with many difficult and complex problems. These difficulties were most visible when approached from the perspective of a lack of effective therapeutic interventions and of societal attitudes toward mental illness. For many years, mental health issues were ignored or, literally, locked in the nation's closets. Deviant behavior was often dealt with harshly, without an appreciation for the underlying diseases causing the behaviors.

While we now recognize that much mental illness is caused by biological factors in the brain, the early history of the mental health field relied on primitive explanations. People whose behavior digressed substantially from prevailing social norms were labeled as witches or deviants. They were viewed through the eyes of a frightened and unenlightened populace. Diagnosis was crude or nonexistent, and therapeutic interventions consisted primarily of various forms of warehousing or, in even worse situations, brutal and inappropriate surgery.

Historically, many mental health patients were allowed to roam homeless. Experts believe that many of today's homeless are mentally ill and in need of care. Hospitals for the mentally ill trace their origins back to the Poor Laws of England in the 1600s and to similar legislation in France.

The formal medical delineation of mental illness did not occur until the late 1800s, when Kraepelin defined various classifications of mental illness. Psychiatry gained great notoriety and, to an extent, legitimacy with the work of Sigmund Freud, who developed many aspects of psychoanalysis. Freud's work related behavior to various unconscious and developmental aspects of personality.

Mental health research and treatments expanded tremendously in the twentieth century. Numerous mental health, mental retardation, and developmental problems were defined and studied. Therapeutic interventions also expanded greatly in the twentieth century. Psychiatric and behavioral interpretations of mind-related problems increasingly used modern medical, social, cultural, and behavioral interpretations.

Many mental health diseases are now known to be biological in origin; these include mental retardation, developmental disabilities, and schizophrenia. Other behaviors are still subject to wider interpretation and professional judgment; these include those related to personality disorders and neurotic behaviors. Defining what is and is not normal in a population is difficult and raises far-reaching moral and ethical issues.

The prevalence of psychiatric problems in our society is difficult to measure accurately. Issues related to sampling, instruments used for measurement, and interpretation of data are especially difficult in mental health. National studies have concluded that among the most common mental disorders are phobias, substance abuse, including alcohol and drug dependence; and affective disorders, including depression. Schizophrenia is considerably less common, affecting perhaps one-half to one percent of the population.

The prevalence of various mental health problems varies for men and women and by age group. Alcoholic drug abuse is the most common impairment for men, while phobias are the most common for women. Depression is also fairly common for women in the reproductive ages.

EARLY MENTAL HEALTH SERVICES

Benjamin Rush is considered the father of American psychiatry. Before the development of formal psychiatric services by pioneers such as Dr. Rush, private medical care was available only to individuals who had financial resources. The early part of the twentieth century was characterized by large, state, inpatient mental health hospitals for the more severely ill.

These institutions warehoused people rather than providing significant therapeutic interventions. The quality of patient life in these facilities, as well as the psychiatric services used to assess patient needs and appropriateness of care, were suspect. The failure to provide adequate psychiatric care has long been a blight on the national health care scene.

The most dramatic development for mental health services in the middle part of the twentieth century was the development of psychopharmacology and psychotropic drugs in the 1950s. These drugs allowed patients to be treated for relatively severe illnesses on an outpatient basis. As a result, beginning approximately in the middle 1950s, the nation experienced extensive deinstitutionalization of some patients from state and local mental health hospitals. Patients with schizophrenia, depression, mania, and other diagnoses were able to be cared for outside of inpatient facilities, using psychotropic drugs.

Censuses of inpatient mental health hospitals declined dramatically. Unfortunately, the care needed for all these patients was not available, and still is not, in community-based settings. As a result, many patients are homeless. Others experience a revolving door syndrome in which they are continually admitted to and discharged from state or local mental health facilities. Patients with insurance coverage or private financial resources may have been cared for in private psychiatric hospitals.

President John F. Kennedy was personally interested in mental health services as a result of his sister's severe mental illness. The Kennedy administration initiated new federal involvement in mental health services, leading to the Mental Retardation Facilities and Community Mental Health Centers Construction Act of 1964.

This act provided construction funds for the development of community mental health services, especially outpatient care. The centers provided care to people without private financial resources. These clinics facilitated continued deinstitutionalization of patients from mental health hospitals. Other facilities, including halfway houses, have also been developed to facilitate the provision of community-based services.

President Jimmy Carter established the President's Commission on Mental Health in 1977, an interest of his wife, Rosalyn. This commission produced a comprehensive report on the status of the nation's mental health system. However, the results of this report were never fully implemented.

The nation has continued to inadequately address its needs for mental health services. Important federal legislation affecting mental health patients is the Americans with Disabilities Act (PL 101–336). This legislation is designed as a civil rights act to protect individuals with physical or mental health problems.

The results of years of biomedical research have substantially increased the armament of drugs available for the treatment of various psychiatric problems. The promise of these new developments, and of even more significant research results in the biomedical pipeline, will require an effective delivery system for patient care dealing with both inpatient and outpatient needs as well as for social and emotional support.

The nation is making significant progress in addressing mental health needs, although resources available in this sector, particularly in the public domain, remain inadequate. Changes in political and public attitudes, facilitated by the development of new treatment interventions and more precise definitions of mental illness diagnoses combined with physiological ideologies have greatly improved the situation. Existing law to encourage greater insurance coverage of mental health services has also provided a positive stimulus, although this legislation has not been fully implemented as yet. The mental health services field, although having a lot of catching up to do, is poised for a number of significant leaps forward, many of which are underway.

MENTAL HEALTH PROVIDER ORGANIZATIONS

Mental health services are provided through public and private resources and both inpatient and outpatient facilities. The nation's mental health system is characterized by two subsystems, one primarily for individuals with insurance coverage or money, and one for those without.

These two complex subsystems, which at times overlap by providing services to a range of patients, include a tremendously broad array of provider organizations. These include, but are not limited to, specialized psychiatric hospitals, as well as acute care general community hospitals; a variety of residential treatment centers for adults, children, and the elderly, including nursing homes, especially those with units specifically oriented toward patients with dementia; outpatient mental health clinics operated by public and private entities; psychiatrists who are physicians with specialty training in mental health services as well as other physicians including internists, family practitioners, and neurologists; psychologists; social workers; and a large component of pharmaceutical industry and associated distribution channels providing inpatient and outpatient drug therapies. The provider networks and organizations are often not well integrated and are separated further by financing mechanisms that segregate mental health organizations, acute somatic medical service organizations, human services agencies, and voluntary agencies. Family and friends also play a key role in mental health support networks, often on a voluntary basis as well.

Patients without insurance coverage or personal financial resources are treated in state and county mental health hospitals, as well as in community mental health clinics. Care is also provided in short-term, acute-care hospitals and emergency rooms.

Local government is the provider of last resort with the ultimate responsibility to provide somatic and mental health services for all citizens regardless of ability to pay. Full implementation of health care reform could substantially alter this picture.

Community-sponsored mental health services are provided to patients without financial resources, often on a sliding-scale, ability-to-pay basis. These services are often provided by psychologists and mental health social workers. The number of Americans in need of care and unable to access even these services is unknown. Other services are also provided in specialized settings for emotionally disturbed children, for those with severe mental retardation, and for the developmentally disabled.

For patients with financial resources, including insurance coverage and the personal ability to pay, there has been a tremendous expansion in availability of both inpatient and ambulatory mental health care. Inpatient mental health services for patients with insurance are usually provided through private psychiatric hospitals. These hospitals can be operated on either a nonprofit or for-profit basis. National chains of for-profit mental health hospitals have expanded over the past 30 years.

Patients with insurance coverage are more likely to be provided care through the offices of private psychiatrists, clinical psychologists, and licensed social workers.

Mental health services are also provided by the Veterans Administration and by military health care. However, access to these services is limited by eligibility.

Managed care is increasingly common in mental health. Insurers are contracting for a limited scope of mental health benefits for enrollees as part of more comprehensive health care packages. Psychiatrists and other mental health providers are contracting with insurers, employers, and managed care plans to provide mental health services for enrolled populations, often based on capitation payments. The ability of managed care plans to provide comprehensive services and to meet the full range of patient needs, given the constraints of these contracts, is an open question at the present time.

An increasingly important component of the nation's mental health needs is care for Alzheimer's patients. As the nation's population is aging, increasing numbers of people, and their families, face the realities of Alzheimer's disease. A wide range of medical and social services is needed to respond to these needs. The development of therapeutic interventions for some aspects of Alzheimer's disease and potential progress from the biomedical research currently being conducted promise a more hopeful future for these patients, assuming that an effective delivery system is in place.

Alcoholic and drug abuse are other serious problems in mental health. Again, the need in the nation exceeds the treatment available in both of these areas.

UTILIZATION OF INPATIENT MENTAL HEALTH SERVICES

Limited data are available on the utilization of state and local mental health facilities. The difficulty of determining the extent to which current national needs are being met complicates interpretation of the data. Mental health services are also subject to variations in interpreting behavior, interventions, and need for services.

Deinstitutionalization and the increasing use of psychotropic drugs did lead to a fundamental shift in the delivery of mental health services for treatable situations. The shift of patients from the inpatient arena to outpatient services was dramatic, and the increasing availability of newer pharmacological agents today is enhancing and reinforcing this shift. However, since the initiation of deinstitutionalization, adequate support and financial resources for providing mental health services on an outpatient basis in communities have often been missing. Today, inpatient mental health services are utilized on a long-term basis for individuals with severe mental health diagnoses such as congenital brain problems, severe accidents leading to neurological deficits, severe dementias, severe retardation, and what historically has been termed acute forms of psychosis that cannot be managed on an outpatient basis. Inpatient services are also utilized for comprehensive intervention for drug and alcohol abuse; episodes of severe anxiety, depression, and other types of urgent mental health needs; and certain other situations. The intent of these episodes of inpatient service is to provide the patient with a platform on which to reenter the family and community environment. Biomedical research is unlikely to ever provide cures for the most severe forms of mental illness, organic brain disease, and severe developmental disabilities. Better prenatal risk assessment and preventive services during pregnancy may help reduce the eventual need for these types of services for many individuals. Preventive services directed toward avoiding the occurrence of mental illness in individuals is tremendously important for the future of national policy in this area. These preventive issues range from protecting the fetus from external assaults that may lead to organic brain diseases all the way to providing healthier work and living environments and supporting family structures for individuals, especially children.

MENTAL HEALTH PERSONNEL

Unlike many other areas of the health care system, mental health services involve many interesting, and sometimes conflicting, personnel issues. Mental health services are provided by a variety of professionals. Patient characteristics, especially the ability to pay, often affect who the provider is.

Psychiatry is the branch of medicine that specializes in mental disorders. Psychiatrists are physicians who receive postgraduate specialty training after medical school in mental health. Psychiatric residencies cover medical as well as behavioral diagnoses and treatments. A relatively small proportion of the total mental health work force is made up of psychiatrists. Psychiatrists exert disproportionate power in the system because they are physicians and can prescribe drugs and admit patients to hospitals.

Psychologists are usually PhDs, although some hold master's degrees. They are trained in interpreting and changing the behavior of people. Psychologists cannot prescribe drugs. The increasing use of psychotropic drugs in the treatment of mental disorders is likely to give greater power to psychiatrists in the future.

However, psychologists provide a wide range of services to patients with neurotic and behavioral problems. Psychologists use psychotherapy and counseling. Psychoanalysis is a subspecialty in mental health, using intensive treatment that is provided by both psychiatrists and psychologists.

Social workers also receive training in various aspects of mental health services, particularly counseling. These social workers are trained at the master's level. Social workers also compete with psychologists and, to a lesser extent, psychiatrists for patients in the treatment of psychological problems.

Nurses are involved in mental health through the subspecialty of psychiatric nursing. Specialty training for nurses had its origins in the latter part of the 1800s. Nurses provide a wide range of services.

Competition among various professional specialties in the mental health arena is also affected by sources of payment. Psychiatrists are more likely to treat privately paying patients and those with insurance; psychologists and social workers are more likely to be prominent public-sector providers. Changes in national financing for mental health could substantially affect competition among these professional groups. The need for therapies for neurotic and personality disorders will remain great for the foreseeable future.

Finally, many other health care professionals contribute to the array of available services. These include marriage and family counselors, recreational therapists, and vocational counselors. Numerous people work in related areas, such as patient day care, alcohol and drug abuse counseling, and as psychiatric aides in institutional settings.

Since mental health impinges on the border between health care and social services, a broad perspective is appropriate. Social workers, police, firemen, social and welfare counselors, and many others in our society are all trying to improve the mental health of our citizens.

LEGAL ISSUES

The nation's legal system has long been involved in the mental health field. The courts have addressed the protection of rights for patients who are institutionalized. The rights of children have also been addressed.

In brief, the courts have ruled that institutionalization without treatment is not permissible. Individuals have a right to care that matches their needs and that is provided in appropriate facilities. Confidentiality has also been addressed, especially the trade-off between confidentiality and threats to other persons.

Advocacy for the mentally ill has gained momentum over the past 30 years. The recognition that much mental illness has biological origins will probably increase individuals' protections under the law.

A responsible and just mental health system needs guidance from the courts and legislatures on many complex issues. People with mental health problems need to be protected. The rights of individuals must be balanced against the needs of society.

PAYING FOR MENTAL HEALTH SERVICES

From a payment perspective, mental health services fall into two major categories: patients who have financial resources, including insurance coverage, and those who do not. Most private insurance pays for some mental health services. Mental health service coverage is often limited to a maximum number of visits per year. Significant copayments by enrollees may be required. Increasingly, managed care contracting is used in mental health, as discussed further later, with provider organizations caring for populations of insured under capitation arrangements.

Public entitlement programs, particularly Medicare and Medicaid, have limitations on coverage. Patients who need care beyond their benefits may first have to use up their own financial resources before becoming eligible for public services. As the provider of last resort, local government is ultimately responsible for providing care to all citizens.

Coverage for inpatient and mental health services expanded during the period from 1960 through the middle of the 1980s. Coverage of inpatient psychiatric care and of alcohol and drug abuse also increased during this period. Some insurance plans have reassessed the nature of these benefits as a cost-containment move. Since mental illness can be quite dysfunctional, limitations on services may be counterproductive.

Providing mental health services is expensive, especially for long-term inpatient care and for treatment of dementia and many other specific categories of mental health service. In addition to the direct cost of services in mental health, considerable costs are associated with the societal and family impact of individuals needing or receiving mental health services. Excellent examples of this impact include substance abuse, including drug and alcohol treatment, and services pertaining to family violence, abuse, and marital discord. Again, the intersection of mental health and social services is a serious issue for coordinating care and financing services. Related and difficult to measure costs include loss of employment time, reduced effectiveness on the job, family and workplace violence, vehicular accidents at least partially attributable to mental health issues, societal violence in general, poor school performance, and on and on.

Comprehensive studies of the global costs of mental health services in our society, extending beyond purely the delivery of health care, suggest a tremendous overall impact for these disorders. Also, potentially included in the computation would be some portion of operating the criminal justice and prison systems, family courts, child social services, and many other related institutions of our society. Prevention, as noted previously, has the potential for tremendous payback but is difficult to implement, particularly for individuals not committing a crime or seeking help as a result of self-referral or family encouragement. In addition, preventive services are rarely paid for directly by any existing payment mechanism; this is especially true of broader preventive issues related to societal violence and interpersonal relations.

About half of all mental health services in the United States are paid for through government programs such as Medicare and Medicaid or direct spending by local government. The remainder of mental health costs are covered about evenly between private insurance and individual out-of-pocket payments or other individual sources. Social services related to mental health are paid for out of non-health care funds by local government or, in some instances, state programs.

In 1996, the Congress passed the Federal Mental Health Parity Act. This legislation was intended to place mental health benefits on parity with other health services. Although legislation has not achieved its original intention, and has many loopholes, some of which have been closed in the intervening years, mental health services are moving closer to parity in the policy arena and in actual practice in some health plans. The potential for extensive utilization of these services with relatively more liberal benefits raises substantial cost concerns. Moral hazard, which is an insurance concept that suggests that increased utilization will be associated with lower cost barriers, is a particular concern in mental health owing to the wide range of potential diagnoses, to self-referral, and to the difficulty in achieving satisfactory closure in treating individual cases. In some insurance plans, the supervising physician or primary care physician may be provided with the authority to control utilization as a means to control costs as well. Similarly, the causes of adverse selection, in that individuals with mental health issues and problems are more likely to select plans that have broader coverage, is a further concern on the part of insurers. Particularly for individuals with long-term and more complex disorders, the potential cost implications to such health plans could be substantial. Many individuals with mental health problems also have increased somatic illness as well, thus increasing overall health care utilization. Thus, financing for mental health services is exceedingly complex and presents many concerns with regard to excessive utilization, definitive diagnosis, accurate and effective interventions, and connection to other health and social services needs.

Ultimately, we need to address directly, particularly during the debates on health care reform, what services should be available and to whom. The increasing ability of mental health professionals to intervene will promote greater coverage. Insurer hesitation in covering mental health services is based on the frequent absence of definitive diagnoses and on open-ended interventions and, often, an inability to cure. As these traits of mental health fade into memory, the scope of benefits should expand.

MANAGED CARE FOR MENTAL HEALTH SERVICES

In recent years, mental health services have increasingly been provided using the mechanisms of managed care. It has become particularly fashionable for managed care companies, and for health care provider organizations that assume responsibility for populations under managed care contracts, to contract with mental health care organizations for those specific services related to mental health within insurance plans. In addition, the locus of mental health services has increasingly shifted to pharmacological intervention with a relatively limited number of clinical visits, and with an emphasis on limited, short-term psychotherapy.

Capitated mental health services have typically involved per member per month payments to managed mental health companies in return for which these organizations provide all covered services. The introduction of capitation, with its associated shifting of risk and reward to the mental health company, changes the fundamental financial arrangements under which mental health services are typically provided. As a result there has been a shift in treatment focus in some situations away from longer-term psychotherapy and toward short-term interventions and use of drugs.

Assuring the adequacy and appropriateness of care is a particularly complex and important issue. The role of psychiatrists, psychologists, and other providers may also be at risk with the emphasis on drug-based intervention and shorter-term therapies. The whole area of mental health services is, of course, being dramatically affected by the increasing identification of biological factors in the etiology of various forms of mental illness, and by the development of new forms of pharmacological intervention for many diagnoses. Cost-containment pressures on the health care system overall are also impinging on the evolution of mental health care in the United States.

Managed care mechanisms in mental health provide an opportunity to contain costs, to standardize treatments, and to provide a greater degree of accountability with respect to provider activity and patient outcomes. Managed care likely also leads to increased utilization of ambulatory as opposed to in-patient services. At the same time, the introduction of managed care payment mechanisms in mental health services raises a number of significant concerns. Inherent tendencies under managed care to provide less rather than more care may lead to underutilization of services.

Sometimes, in the mental health arena, determining the extent of patient need is particularly difficult and subject to provider discretion. These complexities may be exacerbated by payment mechanisms. Treatment modalities may be more specifically prescribed, leading to less provider discretion and perhaps even poorer outcomes. Managed care also often restricts access and patient choice, further complicating patients' initiatives to seek what may be more appropriate care sources. Patient provider interaction is especially important in many areas of mental health services, so this is a fairly significant concern. Managed care organizations may utilize treatment monitoring approaches and outcome measures that are not ideal for certain patients. Treatment modalities may not be appropriate for all patients and may not be individualized to the extent desirable. Mental health providers themselves may find that their practices are dramatically affected by managed care contracts, which in turn determine the numbers of patients they see and the modalities of treatment they apply.

Managed mental health has spread from the private insurance industry to government programs, particularly for services offered under some state Medicaid plans. Managed care for mental health, as for other services, has payer advantages including the potential for prospective budgeting as well as increased cost containment and access controls. The range and complexity of mental health diagnoses often requires that services provided on a managed care basis be carefully defined as to patient characteristics and diagnoses. While managed mental health services have generally been cost effective, applying these principles to individuals with severe long-term systemic mental illness is quite complex. A further complexity is compliance with federal privacy regulations. Contractual arrangements in mental health especially have to be reassessed to ensure patient privacy.

An increased emphasis has also emerged to further integrate mental health services with other care, particularly for somatic illness. Increased integration in part is a reflection of the policy movement to treat mental health services similarly to other types of health care. In addition, the increased application of a medical model and the use of pharmaceutical products to treat mental illness have enhanced this trend.

The long-term efficacy and patient impact of these changes have yet to be fully determined. In addition, many individuals with more serious forms of mental illness are not directly affected by managed care interventions. The increased emphasis on outpatient or ambulatory treatment and reductions in utilization of specialized inpatient mental health services for some patients are other areas for which longer-term analysis is essential.

Other complex issues related to managed care and mental health services include further delineation of the linkage between mental health and other health care services; assurance of confidentiality, particularly with the increased use of computer systems and data analysis to manage the care process; and the determination of which providers will be involved in each aspect of mental health care.

Clearly, increased effectiveness and efficiency and improved integration of care is a benefit long needed in mental health services. Managed care, however, also introduces many other complex considerations in the provision of mental health services. Our nation is in the early stages of the use of managed care in mental health services and the long-term impact has yet to be determined.

THE FUTURE OF MENTAL AND BEHAVIORAL HEALTH SERVICES

Changing definitions and diagnostic criteria have always been characteristics of behavioral and mental health. But over the past 2 decades, the acceleration of biomedical knowledge related to the origins of mental health problems has been even more dramatic than in the past. Definitions of various types of mental illnesses are changing rapidly. In most instances, greater accuracy attributable to a more sophisticated understanding of the biological processes associated with various disease entities has been achieved. Improved and more accurate definitions of diagnostic categories, combined with more definitive intervention, will lead to greater acceptance of these services and improved insurance coverage as well. Entitlement programs, likewise, will be more amenable to coverage for these illnesses as they gain greater legitimacy.

Of course, as in the past, there are many interactions between mental health and other aspects of our society. Criminal behavior, the effects of aging, and behavioral expectations all impact interpretations of various types of mental health. The intricate interaction between illness and culture will always affect interpretations of people's apparent or interpreted health care needs, particularly with regard to mental health.

At the other extreme, with more severe mental health problems, our society needs to recognize the ongoing and fundamental needs of patients whose difficulties are so substantial that their interaction with society will always be impacted. For these patients, biomedical intervention is likely to be of less importance than the creation of an acceptable living environment that reflects humane treatment and some degree of medical intervention. The high cost of providing services for individuals with severe mental health problems will continue to be a burden for our society, particularly with regard to social services spending.

Issues associated with the process of deinstitutionalization still remain a concern. Adequate ambulatory care services have never been developed in some communities. The needs of those individuals subsequently made homeless or patients experiencing the revolving door syndrome must still be better addressed.

The interaction of mental health needs with other problems in our society, such as alcohol and drug abuse, violence, and suicide, also remains a complex challenge. Indeed the social challenges in these areas in the long term may be much more difficult to address than the medical challenges. Balancing societal needs versus individual needs and addressing the complex legal, ethical, moral, and social implications of these very far-reaching problems will be a challenge for the country in the foreseeable future.

In recent years, the political environment for mental health has improved with the increasing recognition of the biological origins of many forms of mental illness. Significant movement to address the treatment of mental illness as a somatic illness has gained ground. National legislation such as the Americans with Disabilities Act and other efforts at the federal, state, and local levels, combined with rapid biomedical progress, holds out hope for a much more enlightened future for mental health services.

Solving the nation's mental health delivery crisis will not be an easy task. Numerous complex issues pertain to the identification and provision of services to patients in need of care, and to the management of those services. Mental health services have long been viewed separately from somatic care, leading to fragmentation in the delivery of services. The integration of mental health and social services, as well as addressing the many relationships between mental health and other aspects of society, such as the work environment, the home environment, relationships, raising of children, schooling,

and the criminal justice system, is a tremendous challenge in and of itself.

The traditional stigma associated with mental health services, although greatly reduced over the past 20 years, still remains a challenge in removing barriers to care and encouraging individuals to seek appropriate help. Lack of adequate availability of mental health services, facilities, and professionals in some geographic areas is a concern. Constraints that still exist, which are substantial, in financing of mental health services for both the private and public sectors are another great challenge. Inadequate recognition of the role of the primary care physician; establishing avenues for appropriate referral for inpatient and outpatient specialty services; addressing cultural, language, and age-related sensitivities in mental health; and the lack of adequate dissemination of knowledge about diagnosis, treatments, and interventions are all further problems that must be addressed. And, ultimately, enhancing prevention throughout out society, not just in the health care system, but also in the workplace, in the family environment, in the schools, and elsewhere, is critical to improving the level of mental health and avoiding the consequences of some types of illness.

Mental health has had a long, tortured history. This has not been a field in which our nation's attitudes and solutions have been adequate to meet our needs. We must hope that the future will be very different from the past.

The increasing success of researchers in identifying physiologic mechanisms for many mental and behavioral problems and in developing pharmacological interventions will greatly improve attitudes toward mental illness. Insurance coverage, acceptance of patients in their communities, protection under the law, and other aspects of mental health issues will be rewarded with greatly enlightened attitudes.

We will still face profound challenges in mental retardation, developmental disabilities, drug, alcohol, and tobacco abuse, violence, and other mental and behavioral problems. The more effectively mental health services reach individuals with such needs, the more harmonious our society will be.

Our society's problems must be faced head on. We need more biomedical research and better health care delivery systems. Problems must be identified, addressed, and resolved. We will all benefit by taking an aggressive and positive stance on behalf of all of our citizens.

STUDY QUESTIONS

1. How did mental health services evolve in the United States during the twentieth century?
2. What are the differences between the public and private sectors in the delivery of mental health services?
3. What has been the history of deinstitutionalization in the United States, and what are its implications for the American population?
4. What are the problems that have occurred in the financing of mental health services?
5. What are the differences among psychiatrists, psychologists, and social workers, all of whom provide mental health services?
6. What are the legal and ethical issues involved in providing health care services in the mental health arena?
7. What has been the impact of psychotropic drugs on the delivery of mental health care in the United States?
8. What is the likely future course of mental health services in the United States?

✑ CHAPTER 8 ✑

Long-Term Care Services

Chapter Objectives

1. To describe the continuum of care for long-term care services.
2. To describe specific services provided within the continuum.
3. To report the role of the nursing home in the delivery of care.
4. To identify who needs and uses long-term care services.
5. To discuss newer forms of long-term care, particularly home health services and hospice care.
6. To relate the key importance of managing, integrating, and coordinating long-term care services.
7. To depict the relationship between long-term care health services and social services in our society.
8. To explore the issues associated with financing of long-term care, including long-term care insurance.

Long-term care services, like mental health services, have been challenged by serious political, economic, and social forces that have inhibited the development and delivery of comprehensive care to our nation's population. Long-term care services include a broad spectrum of care, generally utilized by individuals with severe medical and social problems that limit normal residential living. The complexity of long-term care services and their interaction with other needs create a difficult environment for deciding how best to provide and pay for such care.

Long-term care services are also frequently complicated by the intersection of physical health, mental health, and social service needs. Particularly for the older population, aging is associated with significant deterioration in one or more of these aspects of health. Indeed, a broad definition of long-term care would include a whole range of medical, social, and support services needed for individuals to support their functioning on physical, mental, and social levels over a longer period of time. Long-term care services are often designed to support the patient rather than care for disease, to enhance function rather than to fundamentally change function, and to integrate a range of social and health services for the benefit of the patient.

Our nation has failed to adequately deal with the needs of the American people for long-term care. The current inadequacies of the system need to be addressed in the context of developing an overall, comprehensive health care system. Although attention has been directed to nursing homes and selected other components of long-term care, it is in the integration of all services in the broad spectrum of long-term care, and the coordination of these services with other health and social support, where our nation's efforts have been the most deficient. With the aging of the American population, the challenges of long-term care are likely to grow even greater, and the need for solutions will become more urgent in the future.

THE SPECTRUM OF LONG-TERM CARE SERVICES

In its broadest context, long-term care includes an armada of services, both health-related and social, that are used to help individuals who are fully or partially impaired in their conduct of daily living activities. These services may be provided to individuals within their own homes or may require an institutional base.

Long-term care services may be needed by individuals with relatively shorter term needs because of an acute episode of illness or serious injury. These individuals will eventually recover and return to their normal community settings, although in the interim, and perhaps for an extended period of time, they may require social, mental, and physical health services. Another primary category of users in the long-term care arena is individuals with serious long-term physical, mental, or social difficulties, particularly those with permanent disabilities or situations whereby they will deteriorate in some combination of capacities over an extended period of time. Included in this category are individuals with severe and permanent physical damage such as spinal cord injury and elderly persons with physical, mental, and social deterioration. These individuals need permanent care to support their physical, mental, and social needs including assistance in the living environment and other social services. Since these individuals represent populations that will need assistance permanently, the longer term nature of their situation and frequently the increasing deterioration of their capacities must be recognized in planning the required levels of intervention.

Although most people think of the nursing home as the primary source of long-term care services, the present reality is that a much broader array of services is brought to bear for the benefit of individuals needing such assistance. Among the fastest growing areas of long-term care, for example, are home health services.

The full range of long-term care services provided in the United States is often termed the *continuum of care*. The modern context within which this phrase is used is designed to encourage a broader and more comprehensive conceptualization of long-term care, recognizing the need to bring to bear to each individual the level of services appropriate to his or her situation. In addition, as an individual's physical, mental, and social conditions change over time, the services needed from the continuum of care will likely also change. Comprehensive integration of the continuum of care and appropriate selection of services for each person's needs are important goals for our nation.

Long-term care services are targeted toward those people who are temporarily or permanently (sometimes referred to as chronically) disabled in one way or another. Disability may be due to physical or mental health problems. Most important is the recognition of the primary objective of long-term care in meeting the needs of those who have functional disabilities, particularly those who are unable to perform the activities of daily living on their own without external assistance. Long-term care services extend far beyond health care, including many social and emotional support services as well.

Long-term care services are used primarily by older individuals, although there is a significant number of young people who need such care as a result of permanent or temporary disability. Chronic diseases, including arthritis and other orthopedic disabilities, Alzheimer's disease, strokes and other cerebrovascular problems, complications of diabetes, and visual impairments, are among the physical conditions that tend to be associated with the need for long-term care assistance.

Measuring functional ability among individuals needing long-term care services is achieved through a variety of mechanisms, including traditional medical measures of disease, function, and mental status. However, since social functioning is so important for individuals in the long-term care arena, another set of measures focuses on practical functional status and is termed the activities of daily living (ADL). These include such items as bathing, dressing, eating, using the toilet, and walking. Another set of more practically oriented activities is sometimes utilized including shopping, bill-paying, communicating by telephone, and performing housework. Often, multiple assessments of patient physical status, including illnesses and functional ability; mental health status, including alertness and awareness; and practical living issues, including ability to care for oneself and to safely and securely function in the home, or other environment, are all assessed. The more comprehensive orientation of long-term care services is a hallmark of this field that reflects much broader sensitivity to viewing the patients' total needs in the living environment.

The use of long-term care services increases substantially with age and also in the presence of multiple health problems. The more recent epidemic of acquired immune deficiency syndrome (AIDS) has also increased demand for long-term care services. Among young people, long-term care services are needed for those with congenital abnormalities that prohibit living in a normal household environment, individuals with various serious diseases, plus a spectrum of people who are the victims of accidents.

The use of long-term care services has also increased owing to social trends in our society. Reliance on traditional family support structures, in particular, has decreased with increased female labor force participation and the decreasing prevalence of the nuclear family.

THE SERVICES OF LONG-TERM CARE

Table 8.1 lists services included in the broad spectrum of long-term care. These services comprise the continuum of care but do not reflect those provided by family and friends, the traditional source of long-term care assistance.

Long-term care services include, of course, institutionally based care, such as skilled nursing facilities, and other inpatient services. Extended care facilities include most traditional nursing homes, although it is important to recognize that Medicare establishes specific definitions for various categories of long-term care providers for purposes of their qualifying for reimbursement.

The second category of long-term care services is acute-care services. These include various hospital inpatient services.

The third category of long-term care is home and community-based services, including physician office, outpatient clinic, and various adult day care and mental health services. Psychological counseling and substance abuse are also often included in this category of noninstitutionalized services.

Home health services include the broad spectrum of social and health services provided to individuals in their own homes. This is, as mentioned previously, a rapidly expanding area of long-term care. Included in this category are traditional home health nursing services as well as more advanced medical care, such as infusion and hospice care, and other health-related services. This category also includes a range of social services, such as Meals on Wheels and homemaker services, designed to facilitate an individual's living in his or her own home.

Outreach services are designed to facilitate contact between long-term care service providers and patients. Outreach includes emergency response systems and screening programs. Patient education and outreach are important components of the continuum of care.

Health promotion programs facilitate prevention and improve living conditions. These services include exercise, recreational, meal, and social service programs, and various support groups provided outside of individuals' homes.

The last category of services in the continuum is housing. Various innovations have improved housing alternatives, particularly for older Americans who need some support services. Included in this category are assisted living and congregate-care

Table 8.1. The Continuum of Care Services

Home Care	Outreach and Linkage	Wellness and Health Promotion
Home health	Screening	Educational programs
Hospice	Information/referral	Recreational and social support
Durable medical equipment	Telephone contact	Volunteer programs
Home-delivered meals	Emergency assistance	Meal programs
Homemaker and personal care	Transportation	**Housing**
Ambulatory Care	**Acute**	Continuing care communities
Physicians' offices and outpatient clinics	Inpatient units	Independent housing
Day hospital	Psychiatric care	Congregate care
Adult day care	Rehabilitation	Family care
Mental health clinic	**Extended**	Family homes
Alcohol and substance abuse	Skilled nursing facilities	Assisted living
	Step-down units	

SOURCE: Adapted from Evashwick, C. J., "The Continuum of Long-Term Care' in Williams, S. J., & Torrens, P. R. Introduction to Health Services, (6th ed.). Clifton Park, NY: Thomson Delmar Learning, 2002.

facilities, as well as retirement communities. The objective of these approaches is to provide an environment in which individuals can be housed with some support services but generally avoiding expensive institutional care.

Among the more creative housing alternatives over the past few years have been comprehensive environments that provide a wide range in intensity of services offered depending on an individual's needs. In such settings, individuals are moved into more intensive environments as the need arises. Many of these arrangements require financial agreements at the front end, in return for which individuals are taken care of, regardless of need, for the rest of their lives.

The Hospital's Role in Long-Term Care

Some of the nation's hospitals are long-term care, inpatient facilities. As opposed to short-stay, acute-care hospitals, these institutions focus on the needs of long-term patients.

Many short-term, acute-care hospitals have increased their involvement in some aspects of long-term care, as well. Hospitals are achieving these goals through the establishment of skilled nursing units within the hospital itself or in associated facilities. Patients requiring longer stays than are appropriate in traditional, short-term, acute-care, inpatient facilities may be transferred to a skilled nursing facility located in, or associated with, the hospital. Managed care has encouraged this trend, with hospitals transferring patients to less intensive, skilled nursing facilities to reduce the total cost of hospitalization.

Another area of considerable hospital activity in long-term care is rehabilitation services. Rehabilitation hospitals have become quite popular recently, and many short-term, acute-care hospitals have developed, or are affiliated with, rehabilitation centers. Workers' compensation health care plans have been an impetus to rehabilitation programs.

THE NURSING HOME

The most common component of long-term care services that people think of is the nursing home. There are, in fact, many different types of nursing homes. Table 8.2 presents selected data on the nation's nursing homes. Nursing homes may be independent, freestanding institutions or may be affiliated with, or owned by, other organizations, including hospitals and multi- institutional systems.

The term *nursing home* is generally used to cover a wide range of institutions, and other terminology, such as *convalescent home*, *retirement center*, and *residential care center* may also be used. Specific, legal categorization of nursing homes is defined by Medicare reimbursement policy. Many popular terms are used somewhat loosely and often their meaning is vague.

The nursing homes listed in Table 8.2 include those that are certified for Medicare reimbursement, as well as others offering services on a pay-as-you-go or on a private, third-party basis. Nursing home facilities typically include some degree of skilled nursing care, as well as bed-and-board support services. Length of stay in the nation's nursing homes varies greatly.

Nursing homes may be owned individually or as part of a chain. The increasing integration of health care services has led to more and more nursing homes being bought by multi-institutional systems. These include hospital-based systems, as well as corporations that own and operate nursing homes exclusively.

Table 8.2. Nursing Homes and Beds: United States, 1976 and 2001

Nursing Homes		Beds	
1976	2001	1976	2001
16,091	16,675	1,298,968	1,779,924

For-profit ownership of nursing homes is historically quite traditional, although many nursing homes originated as relatively small, board-and-care, or limited-skilled nursing facilities. The majority of the nation's nursing homes are owned by for-profit entities at the present time. Other nursing homes are owned and operated as nonprofit organizations or are part of larger, nonprofit systems. A relatively small percentage of the nation's nursing homes is operated by government. About three fourths of the nation's nursing homes are Medicare certified.

Nursing homes typically provide care to the oldest and most frail elderly in our population (Table 8.3). The median age of nursing home residents in the United States is about 85 years of age, and three-fourths of such residents are women, who live longer than men. Nursing home residents typically have multiple physical problems and need assistance in various aspects of daily life. Mental health problems, including Alzheimer's disease and other forms of dementia, are also a significant component of the symptomatology of nursing home residents.

Table 8.3. Nursing Home and Personal Care Home Residents 65 Years of Age and Over, According to Age, Sex, and Race: United States, 1999

Age, Sex, Race	Residents
Age	
All ages, 65+	1,469,500
65–74 years	194,800
75–84 years	517,600
85 years and over	757,100
Sex	
Male	377,800
Female	1,091,700
Race	
White	1,279,600
Black	145,900

Only about half of nursing home residents stay in the facilities for more than one year at a time. Relatively few Americans reside in nursing homes, but by age 85 and above, about 20 percent of the population is resident in a nursing home. The average American has about a 50 percent likelihood of residing in a nursing home at least some time during his or her lifetime. Individuals are institutionalized in nursing homes as a result of physical and/or mental health problems that preclude maintenance in their own homes even with support through various social and health services. In addition, individuals who do not have an adequate support structure of family and friends with whom they can live also find themselves in institutional settings when physical or mental health problems become severe enough to preclude independent living.

The nation's nursing homes face many challenges. Many are proprietary or for profit, having to provide adequate services while often facing serious cost pressures. The patients who are residents of the nation's nursing homes have numerous and multiple health care problems and require a high level of maintenance and homemaker services. While some nursing homes are part of larger horizontally or vertically integrated organizations, and thus benefit from efficiencies of scale, many are not. Many nursing home patients receive care paid for by the Medicaid program, which is under tremendous fiscal pressure, particularly since the overheated economy of the late 1990s deflated. Even under the federal Medicare program, which pays for a relatively small percentage of nursing home care (about 25 percent), cost pressures have increased with enhanced emphasis on case mix as a determination of payment levels.

Nursing homes also face regulatory pressures. Previous concerns over quality of care have led to state-administered regulation of nursing home licensure that involves facility inspections with an associated complex survey process and other reporting requirements and supervisory perspectives. On a voluntary basis nursing homes may be accredited by the Joint Commission on Accreditation of Health Care Organizations, but the burden of meeting the necessary criteria is quite substantial, such that not all nursing homes seek this accreditation.

Staff training and turnover are also important considerations in the nursing home environment. The difficult patient mix and cost containment pressures combine with the need for constant frontline housekeeping care to present a high level of stress for employees. Much of the work in nursing homes is performed by low-paid, insufficiently trained direct care workers in understaffed facilities with limited supervisory or managerial personnel available for decision making. Employee stress levels are high while the demands from payers, patients, and families for quality care are intense.

Increasingly, nursing home patients are more and more debilitated, both mentally and physically. Ironically, with the population aging and the quality of life improving for most people, those who end up in an institutional setting are likely to be sicker and more dependent. The increasing prevalence of Alzheimer's disease and other forms of dementia and mental illness further stresses the situation.

Projections of the nation's nursing home needs is not a simple matter. Increasing technology and disease prevention combined with alternative living arrangements may lead to less reliance on the nursing home for future patients as compared to the past. At the same time more people will be living longer, and the result may be a continuation of the current levels of demand, or even increased demand for these services. What will not change easily is the increasing stress for employees and the continuing financial pressures on patients (and their families) who do need nursing home care.

HOME HEALTH CARE SERVICES

Home health care is growing rapidly. A number of large, national, for-profit companies have successfully expanded into this field in recent years. With its cost and social advantages, and with increasing Medicare coverage of such care, home health offers many advantages to patients and payers. Home health is consistent with the philosophy of maintaining people in the least complex environment possible. Few people would prefer institutionalization over living at home. Home health and social services can go a long way toward facilitating this national goal.

Home health care increasingly represents a broader and broader array of services including physical, occupational, speech, and respiratory therapies; social services; case management; patient education; nutrition counseling; and administration of pharmaceutical products. At the other end of the scale, more homemaker and personal care services are also being provided in the home including dressing and personal care, bathing and grooming, transportation, housekeeping, meal preparation, and meal delivery. The increasing array of services provided under the general category of home health is a tremendous asset to patient well being and to reducing reliance on institutional care. At the same time serious issues exist with regard to financing, controlling, monitoring, and evaluating the need for these services for each patient.

Home health services are provided by a wide range of agencies and organizations such as visiting nurse agencies, public organizations such as health departments, for-profit home health care and homemaker agencies, and the range of not-for-profit and community-based voluntary agencies including churches and service organizations. Hospitals, nursing homes, and other health care organizations are also frequently involved in the provision of some of these services. The growth of home health services is limited not by technology, but by payment mechanisms and economic concerns, and by regulatory constraints. In the future, such services are likely to receive considerable attention and potential expansion given their many advantages and appeal to patients and families.

Technological advances allow services formerly provided in a hospital or nursing home to be provided in the patient's home. These services include the administration of intravenous antibiotics, oncology therapies, and intravenous nutrients.

Homemaker services offered in the home are primarily social rather than related to health care. These services greatly facilitate individuals' living at home. Homemaker services include personal care, such as bathing and grooming, meal preparation, transportation, and housekeeping.

As for nursing homes, home health agencies must be certified to receive Medicare reimbursement and, like nursing homes, home health agencies are licensed by the states.

Durable medical equipment (DME) is also provided to patients in their own homes, including the provision of equipment necessary for patient maintenance. Examples of such equipment include specialized hospital beds, infusion pumps, walkers, and oxygen tanks. Again, the objective of these services is to provide what the patient needs in his or her own home and to avoid institutionalization. Most DME providers are for-profit entities.

HOSPICE CARE

Hospice is a concept originally developed in Great Britain to serve the needs of terminally ill patients. The objective of hospice is to provide a high-quality, dignified, and compassionate setting and array of services for patients with terminal illness. Hospice services can be provided in an inpatient, institutional setting or in the patient's home. The hospice concept has grown greatly in the United States in recent decades.

Hospice services include the following: medical and nursing care to patients, both in their homes and in institutional settings, depending on which is more appropriate; homemaker services; inpatient care as needed; therapeutic intervention for the relief of physical symptoms, particularly pain; psychological, social, and emotional support; compassionate consideration for the family; and bereavement services after the patient's death.

Hospice is designed to provide care using a team approach. Respite care is also offered to give family members a break from caregiving duties. Hospice is committed to providing care to the patient and his or her family in a comprehensive manner and considering a much broader array of social and emotional needs than is traditionally found in most health care settings.

Some hospice programs work exclusively through outpatient settings, including the patient's home. Other hospice organizations operate inpatient facilities along with home-based care. Medicare covers hospice services for certain terminally ill patients.

Hospice services are paid for by the Medicare program for a limited time (usually 6 months) in accredited or certified facilities when physician certified. Private insurance typically pays for these services as well. Care provided through hospice programs, particularly by Medicare and private health insurance, covers a broader spectrum of services than is traditionally paid for by health insurance, or by the Medicare program. This is designed to provide sympathetic and comprehensive coverage for patients with terminal illness in a setting that offers more than just pure clinical medical services. This is an exception to the rule that Medicare and private health insurance pay only for medically necessary somatic services and not for a broader array of social services.

COORDINATING THE SYSTEM

Long-term care, with its complex interrelationships between medical and social services, requires more sophisticated integrating mechanisms than many other areas of health care. Services need to be matched to a patient's specific needs, and these needs likely will change over time. Mechanisms for coordinating long-term care services include case management in which a coordinator, sometimes based in a hospital or other setting, identifies patient needs and finds the most appropriate resources in the community. Case management is particularly effective for severe illnesses requiring many types of services.

Management information systems are necessary to support the integration of long-term care services. Linkages between various agencies and government units are particularly important. Since these services cross between health and social services, difficult administrative problems may be involved in paying for care.

Financing of the continuum of long-term care remains a major barrier in providing the full range of services that patients need. Coverage for long-term care, particularly nursing home services, is severely limited under Medicare. In the current environment, individuals are expected to spend down most of their assets in order to qualify for coverage under state Medicaid programs.

Our nation has failed to adequately address issues of financing for long-term care. Social services needed by long-term care patients are generally not included under the health rubric of various entitlement programs. Social services may not be covered at all, particularly for those who are not financially indigent, even though such services may allow individuals to remain in their homes rather than be placed in an institutional setting.

Adult daycare, which is analogous to child daycare, is an excellent example of addressing social but not medical needs in the long-term care arena. Increasingly popular and paid for primarily out-of-pocket and by public programs, adult daycare allows many primarily older or disabled individuals to live with family or with others while being attended to in a caring and responsive environment during the day. However, such services are not viewed as medically necessary and are not integrated directly into health insurance plans and programs. Some

long-term care plans will pay for some of these services.

Integration of social and health services funding is totally inadequate. As a result of the lack of integration and the lack of a coherent approach to financing the complete spectrum of services contained in the continuum of care, management controls, utilization reviews, and the ability to marshal resources are not well coordinated.

Various experimental approaches to improving the integration of the delivery and financing of long-term care services have been attempted. These include social health maintenance organizations (S/HMOs). Other nations, however, have often been at the forefront of innovation in coordinating and integrating services.

The financing of long-term care services remains a complex and essentially unresolved issue for this nation. Until financing issues are adequately addressed, it will be very difficult to provide an efficient and comprehensive framework within which all necessary services can be provided, managed, and coordinated.

Policy and Financing Trends

Funding for long-term care, especially for the nursing home, currently accounts for approximately 8 percent of national health care expenditures. As the average age of the population continues to increase, particularly with an increasing percentage of the population in older age groups, demand for long-term care and nursing home services will be increasing. Political pressures will also build to provide a more substantial mechanism for funding long-term care services, particularly to reduce the extent to which individuals must forfeit their life savings to pay for such care.

An important development in funding for long-term care services is the availability of long-term care insurance. Long-term care insurance is typically applicable to the middle-class population, since the very wealthy can self-fund their needs and the very poor rely on public programs and, in any event, would not have the resources to purchase such insurance. Long-term care insurance is purchased by individuals long before their anticipated need to utilize such insurance. Only physically and mentally healthy individuals qualify for the purchase of long-term care insurance since the insurance companies writing such policies must protect against adverse risk selection. These policies typically cover nursing home, assisted living, adult daycare, home health, and other related long-term care needs, sometimes including care management and usually exclusive of medically necessary services that are otherwise covered by private insurance, Medicare, and other plans and programs. Long-term care insurance is priced based on the level of benefits; the age of the insured when initially signing up for the insurance; the exclusion period between the time when need occurs for such coverage and the point at which the coverage begins; inflation factors, since policies are purchased far ahead of need; and the number of years for which coverage can pay for services—typically 3, 5, or 7 years, or an unlimited time. Long-term care insurance can assure individuals that they will have adequate resources to purchase decent quality long-term care, and as appropriate, also conserve some personal assets for their heirs. The quality and sophistication of these policies have improved greatly in recent years, and now even some employers are offering these policies as a group benefit, albeit paid for fully by the employee. Recent federal legislation has encouraged these trends with tax breaks and other policy initiatives.

The absence of national policy and integrated financing mechanisms can also lead to higher costs. For example, as noted earlier, individuals may be institutionalized because of the absence of available, in-home services. Duplication of services and other adverse consequences of poor integration can result. A myriad of federal, state, and local services and programs exist in addition to many privately offered services. Table 8.4 lists some of the federal government programs currently in existence that provide services relevant to the needs of an aging population.

Finally, our nation also lacks adequate mechanisms for evaluating the effectiveness, quality, and outcomes of most of the services contained in the continuum of care. In recent years, increasing emphasis has been placed on measuring performance in this sector of the health care industry. However, the issues involved in outcome measurement are very complex. Separating the effects of health care services from patients' normal courses of disease and life patterns is a great challenge.

Other unresolved issues include inadequate training and pay for many employees in the long-term care field, especially those at the lower end of the pay scale. There is a need to attract well-educated, efficient, and patient-oriented employees to this field.

ISSUES FACING LONG-TERM CARE

As discussed throughout this chapter, long-term care services have presented, and will continue to present, many challenges to our nation. Ultimately, the issues surrounding long-term care may focus more on social and societal factors than on matters related purely to health care delivery.

With the aging of our population, long-term care will become an increasingly important challenge for the future. Furthermore, projections that people will live substantially longer in the United States as biomedical research yields greater clues to the challenges of chronic disease and aging implies that the future of long-term care may be much more complex and affect many more people than in the past. Ultimately, many of the most complex issues and challenges facing us in long-term care may be more oriented toward economic, social, and ethical concerns than anything else. And with the increasing number of older voters, again as our population ages, political pressures to

Table 8.4. Federal Programs and Legislation in Long-Term Care

Program	Years Enacted
Social Security Act	1935
Veterans Administration	1963, 1972, 1975, 1980
Mental Health Acts	1963, 1967, 1971, 1986
Title XVIII (Medicare), Social Security Act	1965
Title XIX (Medicaid), Social Security Act	1965
Older Americans Act	1965
Housing and Urban Development Act	1965, 1974
Developmental Disabilities Services and Facilities Act	1970
Title XVI (Supplemental Security Income), Social Security Act	1972
Rehabilitation Act	1973
Title XX, Social Security Act	1974
Omnibus Budget Reconciliation Act	1987
Medicare Catastrophic Coverage Act	1988 (repealed, 1990)
Americans with Disabilities Act	1990
Patient Self-Determination Act	1991
Family Medical Leave Act	1993
Health Insurance Portability and Accountability Act	1996
Balanced Budget Act	1997
National Caregiver Support Act	2000

SOURCE: Adapted from Evashwick, C.J., "The Continuum of Long-Term Care" in Williams, S.J., & Torrens, P.R. *Introduction to Health Services* (6th ed.). Clifton Park, NY: Thomson Delmar Learning, 2002.

address many of these issues will grow more intense.

Financial pressures, in particular, have always been of major concern in the area of long-term care. It is these pressures, perhaps more than any other factor, that has inhibited greater insurance and Medicare coverage of long-term care needs.

In recent years, the increasing shift of services to home health care and greater coverage of such care by insurance and entitlement programs has led to substantial increases in the cost of home health services. Pressures have built to contain costs in this area. However, this could lead to a shift back to the increasing use of institutional and hence more expensive services. Home health services have also increasingly adapted to a more high-technology ori-

entation, allowing patients to remain at home for care that previously required institutionalization. Balancing the costs and needs in the area of home health care will be a challenge for many years to come.

The aging of the population and increased longevity, in addition to raising concerns about long-term care needs, suggests that a range of supportive and clinical services will be needed to deal with chronic diseases among the elderly. Maintaining function is a high priority for these services. Some of the newer forms of chronic disease, such as dementia, and in particular, Alzheimer's disease, represent particularly significant challenges and suggest the need for early diagnosis and intervention as well as more effective therapeutic methods. Other diseases, such as arthritis, can have significant long-term costs and associated disability, with a variety of social and other practical needs. Biomedical research and therapeutic intervention are needed across a wide spectrum of chronic diseases to promote function even when cure is not attainable.

Many new and more creative approaches to dealing with the physical, social, and emotional aspects of aging are needed. For example, the Eden Alternative is dedicated to eliminating loneliness, helplessness, and boredom through the creation of environmental habitats for older Americans by creating coalitions that improve living environments. Institutional settings are also responding with creative solutions. Wellspring specializes in rehabilitation for individuals who have suffered abusive religious group relationships and organizations. PACE (Program of All Inclusive Care for the Elderly) is an optional Medicare and Medicaid program that focuses on older individuals and provides comprehensive medical and social services at an adult day health center, at home, or in an inpatient facility generally to avoid nursing home stays. An innovator in these types of programs is OnLok Senior Health Services in San Francisco, California. Other innovative programs are also available or in development to provide alternatives for older Americans.

The need for an integration of social services, such as homemaker services, transportation, meal preparation, and personal care needs, into long-term care has been attempted, as noted, on a limited basis. However, the fundamental nature of long-term care suggests that much greater attention must be directed toward integrating social and medical needs in the future. Failure to do so will severely inhibit the success of the effort to provide comprehensive and integrated long-term care services to all individuals who need such care.

Quality of care is difficult to measure in many long-term care settings, but it is another area that requires additional focus. Ensuring that individuals receive adequate care in a humane and caring environment has always been a fundamental tenet of the long-term care system. Measuring the success to which this is achieved and establishing mechanisms to monitor and ensure compliance have been, and will continue to be, challenges for our nation. Integration of consumer rights in the area of long-term care and consideration of the family, as well as the patient, are likely to be important concerns in the future as well.

Medicaid and personal out-of-pocket payments carry the burden of costs for long-term care, particularly for nursing home care. The increasing utilization of long-term care insurance by individuals who already have some financial means does provide some alleviation for these sources of funds. Longer term, however, our nation increasingly faces questions about the adequacy and appropriateness of the current mechanisms for paying for long-term care services. The lack of integration between long-term care and other health and social services is also quite evident at this point. Cost pressures on government programs and individual personal resources are increasingly stressing the system at the same time that provider organizations face higher costs for personnel and other resources. Demands for better quality and quantity of care also are occurring in an almost unobtainable search for long-term care "nirvana."

Affordability and access to the full range of long-term care services are significant and continuing problems as well. Even individuals needing relatively low-cost homemaker services simply to remain out of the institutional environment may have difficulty accessing and paying for those services. Inner cities, rural areas, and socially isolated individuals all face their own unique problems in this regard. An increasing reliance on voluntary social agencies, churches, and other organizations has provided some help, but these entities are often overwhelmed by the challenges they face in this area. Maintaining and motivating frontline staff in long-term care who work for relatively low pay with difficult patients is a further concern in long-term care.

The increasing role of long-term care services suggests that there will be a need to improve the quality and quantity of the workforce available for these services. Many of the services provided in the long-term care arena do not require a high level of education, but do require training and commitment. In many settings, pay has been inadequate and working conditions have also suffered, especially in the stressful institutional environment. Creating a rewarding workplace in the face of the many difficulties encountered by employees in long-term care environments, training individuals to provide high-quality services, and ensuring an adequate supply of personnel will likely be significant challenges in the future.

Ultimately, the need to address financing shortfalls and mechanisms to allocate adequate resources to this area is the most fundamental challenge that our nation faces with regard to its aging population and its social and health needs. Long-term care is an area in which technology often takes a back seat to more pragmatic and commonplace challenges. But the lack of an overall integrated approach, unified financing, and a creative national commitment to the needs of individuals in the long-term arena remains a huge economic, political, and social challenge for the country.

Individuals utilizing the nation's long-term care "system" ultimately need to have opportunities for choosing the services that they regard as the most attractive to them. Care coordinators and other avenues for assisting individuals in making these selections and decisions are critical. Information systems to provide providers, insurers, and consumers with adequate and coordinated information about alternative sources of care and/or individual patient needs would also have great usefulness. Much needs to be done for coordination of services throughout the entire spectrum of long-term care. Further progress in solving medical and mental health challenges for these populations obviously would be of great consequence, as would preventing or reducing the progression of dementia, improving function for spinal cord injuries, improving function for patients with such diseases as arthritis and other disabling

conditions, and ensuring access to new technologies and medications that are developed through our biomedical research efforts.

Although the long-term care field has evolved tremendously over the past 50 years, much greater progress is needed to meet our nation's goals in this area. In the future, it will be important to achieve greater integration between the different components of the continuum of care and between social and health services. Financing mechanisms also must be designed to encourage greater coordination between components of the continuum and, at the same time, to encourage a more efficient and patient-oriented approach.

Although much has been accomplished, much remains to be done. We owe it to our senior citizens, and to those who are seriously incapacitated at younger ages, to put the pieces together in a humane approach to critical patient needs. At the same time, we must promote cost and administrative efficiencies. To do any less would truly diminish the contributions of a very important sector of the health care industry to our national well-being.

STUDY QUESTIONS

1. What services are included under the continuum of care?
2. How can services in the continuum be better coordinated and integrated with other health and social services?
3. What is the role of the nursing home in providing long-term care services?
4. What is the role of the hospital in providing long-term care services?
5. Who needs long-term care services, and why?
6. What is the changing and expanding role of home health services?
7. In what ways is the hospice an innovative concept in long-term care?
8. What are the major financing and policy questions related to long-term care that our nation has yet to adequately address?

CHAPTER 9

The People Who Provide Health Care Services

Chapter Objectives

1. To describe the training and roles of people employed in the health care sector.
2. To explore in detail the role of the physician in the health care system.
3. To examine physician specialization and geographic distribution.
4. To discuss the changing supply of physicians in the United States during the twentieth century.
5. To examine the changing role of the dentist in the health care system.
6. To describe the changing role of the nurse in the health care system.

The health care industry is one of the largest employers in our nation. Over 12 million people work in the industry, comprising about 9 percent of the total work force of the country (Table 9.1). The health care industry is more capital intensive than labor intensive. Thus, a greater percentage of gross domestic product (GDP) is spent on health care than the proportion of employment the industry accounts for. However, the industry employs a highly educated and well-paid work force holding high quality jobs.

There are many job classifications in the health care industry covering a wide spectrum of skills, education, and duties. Many aspects of health care employment are unique in the economy.

This chapter discusses who works in health care and addresses many issues involving the industry's work force. Although many issues are discussed here, it is impossible to cover completely all of the complex issues involving employment in this diverse sector of the economy. The chapter pays particular attention to the training and roles of physicians and nurses.

THE AMERICAN PHYSICIAN

Physicians have always constituted the most powerful group in health care by virtue of their knowledge, their power to command the use of resources, and their relationships with patients. Physicians have had a long and illustrious history throughout modern times. The physician is a healer responsible for alleviating pain and suffering among patients. Physicians have always been respected and paid well for their services.

Although changes in the health care system, particularly under managed care, are now challenging the decision-making authority of physicians, they still retain tremendous economic and political power. Indeed, press coverage of biomedical progress has led consumers to have unrealistic expectations about the ability of physicians to cure illness and disease.

The physician's role has increasingly involved the use of ever more complex technology in the quest for solutions to patients' needs. The old-time family practitioner would travel to the patient's home, carrying his armaments in a small black bag, providing whatever palliative or curative therapy was available at the time. Today's physician works in a setting surrounded by complex technologies and sophisticated support personnel. This increasing demand for knowledge based on specialization has changed the nature of the medical profession itself.

In addition to an increasingly complex role in the provision of clinical services, physicians are also facing a variety of social and economic pressures. While patients expect physicians to apply the latest technology in the quest for the rapid resolution of their medical problems, they also view the crisis in health care costs as at least partially the fault of physicians for not being more price sensitive in the selection of therapies yet, of course, at the same time expecting all of the latest care. Society, through a variety of mechanisms, is also

Table 9.1. Persons Employed in Health Care: United States, Selected Years

Site	1970	1990	2002
	Number of persons in thousands		
All employed civilians	76,805	117,914	136,485
All health service sites	4,246	9,447	12,653
Offices and clinics of physicians	477	1,098	1,907
Offices and clinics of dentists	222	580	740
Offices and clinics of chiropractors	19	90	138
Hospitals	2,690	4,690	5,340
Nursing and personal care facilities	509	1,543	1,942
Other health service sites	330	1,446	2,585
	Percentage of employed civilians		
All health service sites	5.5	8.0	9.3

increasingly holding the physician more accountable for the quantity and quality of care provided and for the economic relationships that exist between physicians, hospitals, insurance companies, government, and other participants in the health care system. Legislative initiatives, particularly those involving the federal Medicare program, have created complex hazards for physicians in the conduct of their medical practices. Employers, insurance companies, and to an extent patients themselves, have increased their expectations of physician clinical competence, compliance with community standards, and the facilitation of patient communication and access. Thus, as medical knowledge advances, the physician's role in the health care system is becoming increasingly complex, not only for direct clinical care but also as it involves wide-ranging societal and patient expectations.

Specialization in Medicine

Among the most important trends in medicine over the past 40 years has been increasing specialization. Table 9.2 lists some of the major specialties in medicine and surgery and the number of active physicians practicing in each specialty by professional activity.

The old-time general practitioner is no longer a key player in today's health care system. General practitioners were primary care physicians who completed their medical education and a 1-year, rotating internship, and then entered practice. However, medical knowledge has expanded so vastly that 1 year of postgraduate education is now inadequate to prepare an individual for clinical practice.

Taking the place of the general practitioner in today's environment are a number of primary care specialties, each requiring 3 or 4 years of residency, or specialty, training after medical school. These specialties include general internal medicine, pediatrics, obstetrics and gynecology, and, more recently, family practice.

Family practitioners, who complete a 3-year residency, receive training in internal medicine, pediatrics, and obstetrics and gynecology. This specialty started about 30 years ago and is committed to treating the family unit. Family practice specifically trains physicians for primary care careers. Family practitioners are the logical successors to the old-time general practitioners.

Considerable controversy exists regarding whether family practitioners are the most appropriate specialists for the primary care role. General internal medicine, pediatrics, and obstetrics and gynecological specialists argue that they have greater in-depth knowledge in each of their respective specialties than do family practitioners, and are therefore more appropriate providers of primary and specialized care. However, the increasing reliance of health maintenance organizations (HMOs) on family practitioners and excellent patient acceptance have greatly facilitated the proliferation of this specialty.

Recognizing the need to change how physicians are educated, many medical schools now introduce medical students to clinical practice in the first year. Greater emphasis is also placed on cross-cultural issues, communication skills, and patient sensitivities.

A newer type of subspecialist is the hospitalist. This physician, typically an internist, works full time in a hospital inpatient unit and provides intensive care for postsurgical and other patients with acute conditions.

The Supply of Physicians

The number of physicians in the United States has increased dramatically over the past 40 years. Table 9.3 illustrates this growth. Three factors account for the increasing number of physicians in the United States. The numbers of medical schools, of students enrolled in each previously existing school, and of or international medical graduates (IMGs), have all increased.

In the 1960s, as part of President Lyndon B. Johnson's "Great Society" initiatives, there was a concerted effort to increase the supply of medical resources available to our nation's population. These efforts included, of course, the development

Table 9.2. Physicians, According to Activity and Place of Medical Education: United States, Selected Years

Activity and Place of Medical Education	1970	1990	2001
	Number of persons in thousands		
Doctors of medicine	334,028	615,421	836,156
Professionally active	310,845	547,310	709,168
Place of medical education			
U.S. medical graduates	256,427	432,884	537,529
Foreign medical graduates	54,418	114,426	171,639
Activity			
Nonfederal	281,334	526,835	693,358
Patient care	255,027	479,547	652,328
Office-based practice	188,924	359,932	514,016
General, family practices	50,816	57,571	70,030
Cardiovascular diseases	3,882	10,670	16,991
Dermatology	2,932	5,996	8,199
Gastroenterology	1,112	5,200	8,905
Internal medicine	22,950	57,799	94,674
Pediatrics	10,310	26,494	44,824
Pulmonary diseases	785	3,659	6,596
General surgery	18,068	24,498	25,632
Obstetrics/gynecology	13,847	25,475	32,582
Ophthalmology	7,627	13,055	15,994
Orthopedic surgery	6,533	14,187	17,829
Otolaryngology	3,914	6,360	7,866
Plastic surgery	1,166	3,835	5,545
Urological surgery	4,273	7,392	8,636
Anesthesiology	7,369	17,789	28,868
Diagnostic radiology	896	9,806	15,596
Emergency medicine	—	8,402	15,823
Neurology	1,192	5,587	9,156
Pathology, anatomical/clinical	2,993	7,269	10,554
Psychiatry	10,078	20,048	25,653
Radiology	5,781	6,056	6,830
Other specialty	12,400	22,784	37,233
Hospital-based practice	66,103	119,615	138,312
Residents, interns	45,840	81,664	92,935
Full-time hospital staff	20,263	37,951	45,377
Other professional activity	26,317	47,288	41,118
Federal	29,501	20,475	20,017
Patient care	23,508	15,632	16,611

Table 9.2. (Continued)

Activity and Place of Medical Education	1970	1990	2001
	Number of persons in thousands		
Hospital-based practice	19,993	14,569	16,611
Residents, interns	5,388	1,725	739
Full-time hospital staff	14,605	12,844	15,872
Other professional activity	5,993	4,843	3,406
Inactive	19,621	52,653	81,520
Not classfied	358	12,678	38,314
Unknown address	3,204	2,780	2,947

of major entitlement programs, including Medicare and Medicaid, which provided financial support for patients to purchase health care services in the community. At the same time, decision makers in the administration felt that the available community health care resources were too limited. Among those resources targeted for major expansion was the supply of medical personnel, including physicians. Other health professions, such as nursing and public health, were also targeted for expansion.

Table 9.3. Active Physicians and Number per 10,000 Population: United States, Selected Years

Year	All Active Physicians	Doctors of Medicine	Doctors of Osteopathy	Active Physicians per 10,000 Population
1950	219,900	209,000	10,900	14.1
1960	259,500	247,300	12,200	14.0
1970	326,500	314,200	12,300	15.6
1980	457,500	440,400	17,100	19.7
1990	589,500	561,400	28,100	23.4
2000	772,296	727,573	44,723	27.8

Note: Data differ slightly from Table 9.2 because of varied sources and the inclusion of osteopathic physicians.

Expansion in the supply of medical personnel was achieved through a multipronged approach, including federal grants, the expansion of health professions schools, and direct financial support for students. Federal and state governments targeted medical schools for significant expansion.

To increase the supply of physicians, federal and many state legislatures appropriated funding for the development of new medical schools. States such as Texas and California increased the number of state-supported medical schools. The federal government used capitation awards to encourage the development of new medical schools as well. Various other programs also provided incentives for the expansion of medical education.

The net result of these efforts was an approximately 50 percent increase in the number of medical schools in the United States (Table 9.4). This expansion of supply was dramatic and costly. These efforts increased the number of medical school graduates, allowing a time lag for development, construction, initial operation, and graduation of the first classes from these schools. Although medical school supply had held steady for a long period of time, increased emphasis on physician training from the 1960s onward revitalized these national resources in a way that had not occurred since the Flexner report in the early 1900s.

Along with an increase in the number of medical schools, many of the same incentives mentioned

Table 9.4. First-Year Enrollment and Graduates of Health Professions Schools and Number of Schools, According to Profession: United States, Selected Years

Year	Medicine	Osteopathy	Registered Nursing (1996) Total	BA Degree	Associate Degree	Diploma	Licensed Practical Nursing	Dentistry	Optometry	Pharmacy	Chiropractic
First-year enrollment											
2001	16,699	2,927	119,205	40,048	72,930	6,227	—	4,327	1,384	8,922	—
Graduates											
1950	5,553	373	25,790	—	—	—	2,828	2,565	961	—	—
1960	7,081	427	30,113	4,136	789	25,188	16,491	3,253	364	3,497	660
1970	8,367	432	43,103	9,069	11,483	22,551	36,456	3,749	445	4,758	642
1980	15,135	1,059	75,523	24,994	36,034	14,495	41,892	5,256	1,073	7,432	2,049
2001	15,778	2,597	68,709	24,832	41,567	2,310	—	4,367	1,310	7,000	—
Schools											
1950	79	6	1,170	—	—	—	85	42	10	—	20
1960	86	6	1,137	172	57	908	661	47	10	76	12
1970	103	7	1,340	267	437	636	1,233	53	11	74	11
1980	126	14	1,385	377	697	311	1,299	60	15	72	14
2001	125	19	1,508	523	876	109	—	54	17	83	—

previously were used to increase the number of graduates from each of the existing schools. Federal capitation grants were based on the number of medical students enrolled and were effective in encouraging the expansion of medical school classes.

The result of this two-pronged effort was to approximately double the number of medical school graduates in the United States annually (Table 9.4). With increasing specialization and expansion of hospital and other resources, these efforts marked a tremendous commitment by our society to medical education.

Public medical schools are heavily subsidized by taxpayers, while private schools have greater reliance on nongovernmental funding. Federal research dollars help support the missions of both public and private medical schools. Federal and state entitlement programs, such as Medicare and Medicaid, also provide clinical income for medical schools, particularly those providing care to older and medically indigent populations.

The third major avenue for increasing the supply of physicians in the United States was an open-door policy that allowed foreign-trained medical graduates to enter the country and eventually to practice medicine and obtain U.S. citizenship. Foreign medical graduates include all individuals, regardless of national origin, who receive their medical education outside of the United States and Canada.

At the peak years of IMG emigration into the United States, in the middle 1970s, 40 percent of medical licenses were issued to graduates of foreign medical schools. These percentages are far in excess of the historical norm. Current national policy has become much more restrictive.

International medical graduates generally, although not exclusively, emigrated from developing countries such as the Philippines, Haiti, India, and from European and Caribbean medical schools. Mexico, as well, was a source of foreign medical graduates, some of whom were United States citizens unable to gain acceptance to U.S. medical schools.

The ethics of one of the world's richest nations syphoning off critical medical specialists from developing countries is a source of concern. International medical graduates are often drawn from the educational and intellectual elite of their countries. Their skills are, of course, sorely needed at home. The economic incentives posed by practicing in the United States were clearly attractive to many of these physicians. The same issues apply to the many thousands of nurses and other professionals attracted to the United States.

In addition to increasing the supply of physicians, federal policy was also directed toward augmenting the nation's medical resources with nonphysician personnel who could extend the capability of the existing supply of physicians. These individuals included MEDEX, originally returning Vietnam medics who were retrained for civilian practice.

Physician extenders, nurse practitioners, and other specialists augment the use of physician resources. It was felt that these nonphysician clinicians could help physicians practice more efficiently and could perform many of the duties of physicians. This would free up the "limited supply" of physicians to perform more sophisticated tasks.

Physician assistants and extenders met with excellent patient acceptance and have provided good quality care, usually under the supervision of a physician. The success of these personnel led HMOs to use them as well. However, increasing competition between physicians and nonphysicians for a limited patient supply is putting strains on the economic viability of these nonphysician providers.

In addition to more physicians with augmented capabilities and better support personnel, there has been enhanced emphasis on efficiency. Practitioners who work more efficiently, seeing more patients per hour, effectively increase specialists' resources.

Physician supply has increased dramatically since the 1960s. In addition, the availability of a wider array of health care resources to augment physician supply has also characterized the past 40 years. For a time, there was general consensus that current and future supply would be adequate overall and for most physician specialties. These assumptions are now being reassessed such that future physician supply may indeed not be as adequate as was earlier anticipated. Many complex factors affect the translation of physician supply to actual clinical practice time. Some physicians attend medical school but then do not practice clinical medicine, rather focusing on other pursuits such as journalism, politics, or even financial services. Many physicians are retiring at an earlier age than previously anticipated, although the financial realities of medical practice these days suggests that this trend will likely taper off soon.

Physician productivity is another huge issue in interpreting the adequacy of physician supply. The ability to see more patients in a clinical work day or to perform surgical or other procedures more efficiently, and thus in a quicker fashion, can substantially increase the utilization of existing medical personnel. A more efficient office practice with better support services and improved scheduling of patients and of clinical time can have a dramatic impact on physician utilization.

The changing nature of disease and illness itself can dramatically impact the need for clinical personnel. The aging of the population and other demographic, social, and economic trends in the larger society also can impact demand for health care services and thus physician requirements. Training physicians is an expensive and time-consuming process requiring long lead times, yet the uncertainty of physician supply requirements for the future makes planning quite an imprecise science. Health care personnel policy in general, and projections of physician needs for the future specifically, are challenging policy areas for our nation.

Characteristics of Medical Students

During the time of the Great Society in the 1960s, federal and state governments also pushed to increase the number of minority and women students enrolled in medical and other health professions schools. Historically, the representation of women and minorities in these professions has been extremely low in comparison to their proportion in the general population. Overt discrimination against women and minorities was probably prevalent in many health professions schools. To rectify these injustices, programs provided financial and academic assistance to qualified women and minorities.

Tables 9.5 and 9.6 present information on the enrollment of women and minorities in medical and other health professions schools. The changing nature of our society, particularly increased participation of women in the labor force, has led to much higher enrollment rates for women in health professions schools.

In past years, female medical students were rare. One medical school was started in Philadelphia solely for the education of women as physicians. Similarly, representation of minorities was extremely limited in the traditional, white-dominated medical schools. A number of medical schools, such as at Howard University, were started to educate black physicians.

Female enrollment in medical schools has increased dramatically. A female applicant to medical school today has the same chance of admission as a comparably qualified male applicant. Barriers to women in residency training and other career pathways in medicine and in other professions have also largely fallen by the wayside. Surgical specialties, except for obstetrics and gynecology, have probably been the least receptive to women. Now, however, women populate all fields of medicine.

The results to date for minorities are less encouraging. Significant underrepresentation still exists for most minority populations, except for Asians.

Table 9.5. Percentage of Minorities in Schools for Selected Health Occupations: United States, Academic Years 1970–71, 2000–01

Occupation	1970–71	2000–01
	Percentage distribution of students	
Dentistry		
All races	100.0	100.0
Not Hispanic or Latino		
White	91.4	64.4
Black or African American	4.5	4.7
Hispanic or Latino	1.0	5.3
American Indian	0.1	0.6
Asian	2.6	25.0
Medicine (Allopathic)		
All races	100.0	100.0
Not Hispanic or Latino		
White	94.3	63.8
Black or African American	3.8	7.4
Hispanic or Latino	0.5	6.4
Mexican	—	2.5
Mainland Puerto Rican	—	0.7
Other Hispanic	—	3.2
American Indian	0.0	0.8
Asian	1.4	20.1
Medicine (Osteopathic)		
All races	100.0	100.0
Not Hispanic or Latino		
White	97.3	76.1
Black or African American	1.2	3.7
Hispanic or Latino	0.8	3.5
American Indian	0.3	0.7
Asian	0.5	16.0
Pharmacy		
All races	100.0	100.0
Not Hispanic or Latino		
White	90.6	58.8
Black or African American	3.7	9.5
Hispanic or Latino	1.4	3.7
American Indian	0.2	0.5
Asian	3.8	20.6

Table 9.6. Total Percentage Enrollment of Women for Selected Health Occupation Schools and by Race for Allopathic Medicine: United States, 1971–72 and 1999–2000

Enrollment, Occupation, Detailed Race, and Hispanic Origin	Women	
	1971–72	1999–2000
Total enrollment	Percentage of students	
Allopathic medicine (all races)	10.9	43.9
Non-Hispanic white	—	41.5
Non-Hispanic black	20.4	62.0
Hispanic	—	45.4
Mexican	9.5	44.0
Mainland Puerto Rican	17.1	48.8
Other Hispanic	—	44.0
American Indian	23.8	47.6
Asian	17.9	44.0
Osteopathic medicine	3.4	40.2
Dentistry	3.1	37.8
Optometry	5.3	53.1
Registered nurses	95.5	87.9

Minority medical school enrollments increased with the strong federal and state training emphasis of the 1960s and early 1970s, but they fell off as these efforts slackened.

With the substantial historical deficiency in minority representation among practitioners, even a very successful effort would take many years to dramatically alter the total practitioner pool. There are still inadequate numbers of minority medical students and graduates and a significant underrepresentation among the pool of providers in clinical practice.

Alleviating enrollment deficiencies for women and minorities has required an examination of the educational pathway. For physicians, this includes a rigorous college education. Potential applicants have to recognize that medicine is a viable career option, something that for years was not visible to most women and minorities.

Applicants from female and minority populations must be motivated to seek entry to medical and other health professions schools. Women deserve access to a full range of professional opportunities and increasing labor force participation. As society has changed, so too have individuals' expectations concerning viable career pathways. For women interested in the health and helping professions, medical school is now recognized as a viable option. In earlier days, women were often channeled by societal values into other, traditionally female, careers.

Societal attitudes toward minorities in the health professions still need improvement. The entire educational pathway has to be geared toward helping people recognize and access the rigorous preparatory education needed for medical and health professions schools. Many challenges remain for our society. With an increasing need for women and minorities to be in community practice, we must continue to address these issues.

GEOGRAPHIC DISTRIBUTION OF PRACTITIONERS

In addition to a perception in the 1960s and 1970s that the total number of physicians was inadequate and that the specialty mix was wrong, problems were identified with the geographic distribution of practitioners throughout the country. In the 1970s and before, there was an inadequate supply of physicians in rural areas and in inner cities. Physicians are attracted to practice in areas where income and cultural, environmental, housing, and medical resources meet their expectations.

Many programs were started to address these problems. One of these was simply to increase the supply of physicians so that some would be forced by economics to practice in traditionally deficient areas. Another approach was to attract to medical schools people who came from underserved areas, expecting them to return "home" after their training. A further approach was to have medical students rotate through inner city and rural areas with the hope that they would find such practice to be attractive. The National Health Service Corps was created as a mechanism for subsidizing medical students' education in exchange for service in medically underserved areas.

Of all these initiatives, the most successful has probably been flooding the country with physicians, leading to a forced improvement in geographic distribution. Although inner cities are still experiencing deficiencies in some parts of the country, many rural areas have seen dramatic increases in the availability of physicians. In addition, the use of nonphysician, midlevel practitioners has also facilitated the availability of medical resources in many of these communities.

THE NURSING PROFESSION

Nursing is a vital profession in health care. Nurses provide extensive clinical services to patients and support the role of the physician. Many nurses assume relatively independent responsibilities for highly complex patient services as well. Nurses also serve an important managerial role in helping to organize and run the health care system.

There are nearly 2 million registered nurses in the United States (Table 9.7). However, many nurses do not work in the health care field, having found better opportunities elsewhere. In addition, the demands for employment at inconvenient times or with inadequate pay have hindered the participation of women in nursing. Few nurses are males. As nursing is a predominantly female occupation, family and child-bearing concerns are often raised.

There are many categories of nurses. Registered nurses obtain an appropriate education, take a state licensing examination, and receive licensure. The education of registered nurses historically has occurred in 3-year diploma programs offered through hospitals. Since the 1980s, baccalaureate degree programs in nursing have gained prominence. Many professional nurses, particularly those

Table 9.7. Active Health Personnel by Occupation: United States, 1999–2000

Occupation	Number of Active Health Personnel
Nutritionists/dieticians	97,000
Occupational therapists	55,000
Physicians	772,296
Federal	19,228
Doctors of medicine	19,110
Doctors of osteopathy	118
Nonfederal	753,068
Doctors of medicine	708,463
Doctors of osteopathy	44,605
Optometrists	29,500
Pharmacists	208,000
Physical therapists	144,000
Registered nurses	2,271,300
Associate and diploma	1,290,400
Baccalaureate	739,000
Master's and doctorate	241,900
Speech therapists	97,000

in nursing education, believe that requiring the baccalaureate degree raises the stature of nursing and improves the quality of care administered.

In addition to diploma and baccalaureate degree programs, nurses can obtain the registered nurse license after completing a 2-year associate degree program. There is little evidence that the quality of nursing education is inadequate in any of the three paths to the registered nurse license. However, the baccalaureate program probably does a better job of training nurses for high-tech positions, while the diploma and associate programs may be better oriented toward frontline nursing.

Considerable attention has been directed toward the shortage of skilled nursing personnel in many areas of the country. For many years, nurses have battled relatively difficult working conditions, long hours, night hours, pay that is relatively inadequate from many perspectives, substantially increasing paperwork load, and many other considerations. Many nurses do not practice nursing but have sought careers in other fields that are viewed as more attractive. For a long time, the United States has imported nursing personnel from other countries around the world. Funds to expand nursing education in the United States have been limited so that it has been difficult to increase the supply of available nurses in many states. Nurses also battle a variety of political and social difficulties, both in working with patients and in dealing with superiors and administrators. Nursing is on the front lines while at the same time is caught in the middle between physicians and patients, between institutions and organizations and patients. Nurses also face the need to keep current; to participate in efforts to reduce medical errors; to adapt to new information collection and evaluation systems; and to meet the needs of managed care organizations, information systems experts, and a host of other concerns ranging from ergonomics to social needs of patients.

Nursing education also encompasses master's and doctoral degree programs. The master's level includes nurse practitioner programs in various specialties. Nurse practitioners provide clinical services, such as well-baby care and primary care. Nurse anesthetists provide considerable obstetrical care. Nurse case managers and administrators provide key roles in clinical care and organizational operations.

In most states, nurse practitioners practice under the supervision of physicians. Nurse practitioners are seeking the right to practice independently. Physicians generally oppose such efforts for competitive and quality reasons. Yet nurse practitioners provide excellent quality care and have achieved high levels of patient satisfaction.

Many complex factors relate to nursing in the United States. Ultimately, nurses are critical to the success of clinical practice and the care process. A supply of well-trained, motivated, and committed nurses is essential for the nation's health care future. Issues such as improving workplace conditions, helping nurses cope with the stress of the clinical environment, providing an adequate and motivating comple-

ment of salary and benefits, and involving nurses in clinical decision-making and quality of care processes and outcomes is essential. Reducing paperwork and streamlining clerical and administrative processes are key to achieving nurse satisfaction as well.

In summary, the nursing field has changed dramatically and is continuing to evolve. Since its origins with Florence Nightingale and other pioneers, nursing has been committed to frontline patient care. With the evolution of technology and the expansion of the health care system, nurses have increasingly sought greater professional autonomy and an expanded role in clinical decision making. The higher levels of education required now in nursing have promoted more professionalism, higher pay, better working conditions, and greater involvement in management.

Cost containment and political and economic crosscurrents in the health care system are exerting pressures on nurses' pay while also increasing responsibilities and limiting independence. In the future, these crosscurrents will continue to play out as the health care system evolves. The future role of the nurse will be determined by many of these interacting forces.

THE DENTIST

Dentistry has been eminently successful over the past 40 years in promoting the health of its clientele. Tremendous strides have been achieved in improving the oral health of the nation's population, particularly for those individuals with adequate access to dental care.

Dentistry has become much more competitive. Increased operational efficiency, particularly with the use of auxiliary personnel, such as dental hygienists, and more advanced technology have further heightened this competition. Finally, the increasing inroads of managed care have further pressured dentists.

Dentistry faces a number of unique and interesting supply versus demand issues as well. With the increased efficiency and productivity have come decreases in demand for dentists, as reflected by reductions in number of dental schools and dental school graduates. At the same time, however, a significant number of individuals in this country do not have adequate access to dental services owing to financial considerations. Since the predominance of dental care is paid for by dental insurance or out-of-pocket by individuals themselves, people who lack financial resources also may lack access to dental care. These individuals represent a significant, unmet need for dental care, but until financial resources are committed through public or other sources, a significant imbalance between supply and evident demand is likely to continue. There is also a huge reservoir of additional potential demand attributable to desires for cosmetic dentistry, need and desire for orthodontia, and other popular expansion areas for dental services.

OTHER HEALTH CARE PERSONNEL AND ISSUES

Many professions are involved in the health care system. There are many complex issues affecting the roles of these professionals and their interaction with other components of the system. For example, ophthalmologists, who are physicians trained in eye care and surgery, optometrists, and opticians compete for certain aspects of the eye care business, such as eye refractions and prescribing glasses and contact lenses.

In pharmacy, the increasing complexity of drugs has heightened the role of pharmacists in patient education and compliance. A massive shift toward managed care contracting in the pharmacy industry has changed the economics of pharmaceuticals. Distribution channels for these products have changed with less focus on traditional retail pharmacies. Mail-order distribution, in particular, has become an important avenue for distribution of drugs.

Physical therapy and occupational therapy are areas that have seen great growth. Workplace injuries and the expansion of rehabilitation services have fueled the growth of this industry.

Many types of professional opportunities are available in the health care field, ranging from those that require relatively little other than on-the-job training to neurosurgery. The changing nature of the technology of health care is constantly creating new job classifications and opportunities as well. The need to augment available resources, such as physicians, also creates opportunities for physician assistants, nurse practitioners, and many other professionals. The huge array of existing technical jobs ranges from dental assistants to program coordinators to pharmacy technicians to coding technicians, and the list is growing longer every day. Computer technologies are expanding rapidly in health care, requiring more systems analysists, programmers, and implementation specialists. Individuals with skills to operate specialized equipment are in particular need, such as for operating room equipment, imaging equipment, computer networks, and security operations. Some of these positions provide opportunities for additional training and advancement, while others have a more limited career track. Some positions have a limited future as technology changes as well. The health care field is both capital and labor intensive, requires constant training and retraining of personnel, and is always evolving and adapting to changes in technology, financing, and operations. In addition, changes in the structure of the system and its financing, such as managed care, introduce further demands on personnel into the system. Individuals who can facilitate greater efficiencies in the system, whose skills might substitute for more expensive alternatives, and who can play a role in better organizing and managing the health care system will also be in demand.

Many health care workers are directly impacted by reimbursement and insurance issues. For example, recent changes in Medicare have decreased payments and quantities of services provided.

Emergency medical care is another growth area. The nation has moved to expand and integrate emergency medical systems in most major cities.

Health services administration has grown tremendously over the past 40 years. Administrative positions are available in hospitals, clinics, and other health care settings, as well as in insurance and managed care companies. Numerous other opportunities exist and new ones are added to the menu of choices each year as the health care system expands in scope. Training is available at the undergraduate and graduate levels for interested individuals. Individuals in clinical and other areas need to acquire the ability to perform multiple tasks; to adapt to changing technology, economics, and community needs; and to respond to the need for new types of allied health professionals as the nature, location, and technology of health care changes.

THE FUTURE OF HEALTH CARE PERSONNEL

The backbone of the nation's health care system is the people who work hard in providing services throughout the system. These people include frontline, hands-on providers, support personnel, administrators, and many behind-the-scenes professionals who make the system function. The people involved in the production and distribution of medical supplies, devices, and therapeutic agents are equally important to the success of health care. The range of health care professions is impressive, and the professional challenges are equally great.

Considerable questions remain as to the appropriate level of supply of physicians necessary to meet the needs of our country. Parallel issues persist with regard to specialty distribution, emphasis on primary versus specialty care, geographic distribution, and needs for auxiliary specialists to complement the existing physician supply.

The dramatic increase in the supply of physicians, as discussed earlier, resulted in dramatic increases in the number of practicing physicians in the United States. Projecting demand, considering such complex issues as effectiveness and efficiency, changing medical technology, and the impact of managed care on cost containment and resource utilization are extremely difficult challenges. Changes in disease patterns, in availability of nonphysician personnel, in the location in which care is provided, and many other factors discussed throughout this book obviously impinge on any analysis of the need for physicians as well.

The increasing focus on primary care physicians is threatening to adversely impact the training and availability of subspecialists in many areas of practice. In the future, with the increasing sophistication of biomedical knowledge that is now occurring, our nation may find itself in the position of having too few subspecialists. Although the consensus is that we need fewer subspecialists, the complex training that they require and the difficulties of expanding such training would suggest that cutting back too far in this area could lead to future problems.

Medical education itself has changed dramatically over the years. Schools are addressing key changes in the nature of health care delivery. Many schools are examining the emphasis that needs to be placed on ambulatory as opposed to traditional inpatient education. The importance of increased emphasis on mental health and other previously underemphasized areas in the undergraduate medical curriculum is being addressed. Educating future physicians about their roles, pressures, and responsibilities when working in a managed care environment is a new topic at many schools.

At the same time, medical education and academic health centers are facing tremendous cost pressures as payers, including government programs, are increasingly reluctant to pay for the costs of medical education. Insurance industry and government policymakers have also sometimes been unwilling to provide funding for research and other academic activities.

Physicians and other health care providers are facing tremendous pressures from other quarters as well. Medical malpractice premiums, particularly in certain parts of the country and in some high-risk specialties, have skyrocketed as a result of the increased litigation by patients who feel that the quality of care that they received was inadequate or inappropriate. The medical malpractice environment is an imperfect stage on which to rectify errors experienced by patients, since many cases of malpractice go uncompensated while others are the subject of huge awards, perhaps out of proportion to the damages suffered. But ultimately, the cost of malpractice insurance, litigation, and settlements is priced into health care throughout the system. Compulsory arbitration and risk management have focused on reducing these costs, but other aspects of malpractice, such as defensive medicine, in which physicians perform tests that may not be necessary primarily to protect themselves against future litigation, also ratchet up the cost of health care services. In addition to the malpractice arena, physicians are increasingly being called to account to a variety of mechanisms, including relicensure and recertification of their specialty credentials, and physician report cards, in which they are evaluated across a variety of criteria. Most larger physician organizations assess the performance of their physicians and other clinicians against preestablished standards to ensure that at least minimum criteria standards are met in clinical practice. Hospitals, of course, have conducted such reviews for many years in various forms, as discussed later in this book. The challenge for all clinical practitioners ultimately trying to do what is best for the patient, which is one thing that most clinicians strongly believe in, and at the same time meeting a variety of political, financial, utilization, and other criteria standards certainly complicates the lives of many of the people working in the health care system today.

Other health professionals, of course, as discussed previously, are also facing numerous complex issues related to their role in the health care system and to their training. Nurses, pharmacists, vision care experts, and many other professionals see a rapidly changing environment in which they strive to define their roles and to ensure their future viability

as health care professionals. Competition for business is increasing. Examples of competition include that between primary care physicians, nurse practitioners, and physician assistants; in mental health between psychologists, psychiatrists, and clinical social workers; in vision care between ophthalmologists, optometrists, and opticians; and in medicine itself between physicians of different specialties.

Most health care professions are also being affected by fundamental changes in the characteristics of individuals seeking training. For example, increases in the number of women participating in most professional categories are probably changing the dynamics of the work environment.

And finally, managed care itself is impacting many types of health personnel. In addition to shifting the financial risk for care to providers, managed care has changed many of the traditional relationships between payer and provider. Managed care organizations are increasingly dictating the patterns of practice adopted by health care professionals and are developing specific clinical indicators of success that can be applied to physicians and other practitioners.

Increased emphasis on cost-effectiveness and efficiency translates into direct changes in the ability of practitioners to practice in the ways they desire. Pressures from managed care are, in turn, translated into pressures on physicians and other practitioners to work more effectively, to spend less time with each patient, and to utilize all resources more carefully. These pressures have dramatically changed the philosophical and pragmatic environment within which practitioners provide health care throughout our nation.

Health care is a difficult field in which to work. The problems faced in the industry are complex. Issues of life and death are faced every day. Economics, social policy, ethics, and politics are constant concerns. The enhancement of the work environment, professional efficiency, and the education of health care professionals must be high priorities for our nation as we move into an increasingly technological and challenging environment for health care.

STUDY QUESTIONS

1. How many people are employed in the health care system, and what do they do?
2. How was the supply of physicians expanded during the latter part of the twentieth century?
3. Where have foreign medical graduates come from, and what are the ethical issues involved in allowing them to practice in the United States?
4. Is there likely to be a surplus of physicians in the United States in the future?
5. What issues are involved in increasing the supply of females and minorities in the medical profession?
6. How has the role of the dentist changed, and what likely future changes will occur?
7. What is the role of today's nurse in providing health care services, and how did that role change in the latter part of the twentieth century?

CHAPTER 10

Research, Technology, and Pharmaceuticals

Chapter Objectives

1. To describe the role of technology in health care.
2. To describe the organization of the pharmaceutical industry.
3. To explain how pharmaceutical regulation operates.
4. To address significant issues facing the nation with regard to pharmaceuticals.

THE ROLE OF TECHNOLOGY AND RESEARCH

The health care system exists for purposes of delivering the biomedical technology that our research scientists have developed over the past 50 or so years. Technology changes dramatically over time, and that means that the health care system itself must also change. The people who provide health care services also must change and adapt to the latest technologies. Curing disease, the success of the nation's health care system, is dependent on our technology.

Technological advances can often be dramatic. For example, the discovery of the germ theory, which led to safe surgical technique, and the introduction of anesthesia dramatically changed our ability to respond to disease. The discovery of penicillin and other early drugs such as antibiotics was equally dramatic in its impact. A third example is the development of X-ray equipment and eventually the identification and development of more sophisticated imaging technologies such as computer-assisted tomography (CAT), magnetic resonance imaging (MRI), and ultrasound that have radically changed the practice of medicine over the years. Technological advances are at the core of the nation's health care system.

The dissemination of knowledge regarding technology and the assimilation of technological advances into the practice of medicine are also important and should be based on objective scientific discovery and clinical analysis. Sometimes technology is not used appropriately and at other times it is underutilized. Thus, the availability of technology does not ensure its appropriate utilization in clinical practice. In addition, the costs of new technology are often high and require reimbursement by payers to allow for widespread use in clinical practice.

Many new and amazing technologies have been developed in recent decades. As a result of basic research, we have a tremendous ability to understand the molecular basis of illness and disease. Genetic research is uncovering the fundamental determinants of human life. In reproductive medicine we have the ability to enable couples to have children where they previously had little hope. We have the ability to replace human joints that wear out, to perform a huge range of complex and sophisticated diagnostic tests to help us understand individual needs for clinical intervention, and are much better able to decipher the biological origins of mental illness. The future of technology is virtually unlimited although the costs involved give us some pause.

THE PHARMACEUTICAL INDUSTRY

In the United States, the pharmaceutical industry is one of the key components of the nation's health care system. Pharmaceuticals are becoming more important to the therapeutic regimens available to physicians and other practitioners in addressing the needs of patients. With the tremendous progress in biomedical knowledge that is now occurring, the pharmaceutical industry will continue to play a key role in the nation's health care system.

The pharmaceutical industry is large and complex. It has evolved over the years into a highly sophisticated array of biomedical research, marketing, production, and distribution components. The industry faces many challenges ranging from the development of new products to political and economic pressures accruing to its key role in product distribution and pricing.

The pharmaceutical industry in the United States operates in a worldwide environment. In addition, many other pharmaceutical companies in other nations distribute products in the United States. Pharmaceuticals transcend international borders and represent a key industry in the increasing globalization of worldwide business. Characterized increasingly by mergers and acquisitions, it is highly likely that the increasing skill achieved through international organizations and worldwide markets will continue to set a pattern for this industry in the future.

The pharmaceutical industry produces products that represent approximately 8 percent of the nation's health care dollar. The pharmaceutical industry also accounts for approximately one half of all biomedical research in the United States. Pharmaceuticals, however, are an increasingly significant therapeutic modality and a focus of substantial biomedical research.

The pharmaceutical industry has been expanding with an increased effort on research, marketing, and distribution. The Internet is increasing the facilitation of these efforts along with enhanced patient education.

Pharmaceutical companies and their related brethren produce pharmacological agents, medical devices, and other products utilized in the provision of health care services. In the broad characterization of this industry, products that are utilized for patient care range from surgical items to over-the-counter drugs.

The pharmaceutical industry is responsible for the research of new products, identification and development of new products, the manufacture and production of those products, and, finally, their marketing and distribution. The pharmaceutical industry includes a wide range of companies, some of which are traditional old-line drug companies, such as Johnson & Johnson, while others are newer biotechnology companies, such as Amgen or Neurocrine Biosciences. Many other companies are also involved in the industry including generic drug manufacturers who produce generic versions of previously patent-protected pharmaceuticals, and a wide range of companies producing medical devices used in the provision of health care services.

Most pharmaceutical companies manufacture their own products in highly regulated settings. Increasingly, the production of pharmaceuticals requires sophisticated technology and extensive quality assurance. Drug delivery mechanisms for the provision of these products to patients has also broadened over the years to include injectables, oral drugs, time-release patches, nasal sprays, and other methods. More direct delivery of many agents allows for a reduction in side effects and for more rapid absorption of the agents by the body.

It is in the area of biomedical research that many drug companies expend tremendous effort. Pharmaceutical companies that develop their own products must constantly invest in research and development to ensure that their pipeline of new products is providing them with innovative and marketable drugs. In addition, as patent protection ends for existing products, new protected products must be brought to the market. It is the newer products that command the highest premiums in the marketplace, since generic drug manufacturers cannot copy and sell the same products.

Historically, biomedical research and particularly pharmacological research has been based on traditional laboratory bench research. In recent years, however, much more sophisticated technology has been applied to pharmacological research utilizing computer-based and automated systems to examine the potential of a large number of compounds for clinical application. In addition, many pharmaceutical companies have merged and consolidated their research efforts to provide a much more substantial investigative effort. Enhanced imaging and measurement equipment has also facilitated the development of new technologies in health care.

Although biomedical research is also heavily supported by the federal government, primarily though the National Institutes of Health, the private pharmaceutical industry has increasingly emphasized the importance of its own efforts. In addition, many old-line pharmaceutical companies have been purchasing other drug companies in order to take advantage of their biomedical research and drug product pipelines.

Many of the larger pharmaceutical companies in the United States and worldwide also produce products for animal health and for other markets. These companies frequently develop and sell products that are sold over the counter for human consumption, such as common pain relievers. In many instances, products that initially begin as prescription drug items eventually evolve into multiline products with over-the-counter components.

Marketing and distribution of pharmacological products is an additional important component of the operations of most drug companies. Historically, prescription drug products in particular were marketed directly to physicians because they had the ability to prescribe these products for their patients. In recent years, however, many drug manufacturing companies have utilized other communication channels to market products directly to consumers. They expect consumers to seek out these products from their physicians or identify these products as more desirable than other products in the market for the same condition. Some controversy exists about the direct marketing of prescription drug products to consumers, but most in the industry consider these efforts to be worthwhile for more popular products.

Marketing to physicians has historically been directed through a number of key channels. Advertising and direct-mail campaigns aimed at physicians, including advertising in medical journals and professional publications, have long been popular avenues for the dissemination of information from pharmaceutical manufacturers to physicians. In addition, drug companies historically have employed marketing representatives (detail people) who meet directly with physicians and other key decision makers to enlighten them about these products. Physician "education" has proven to be a very effective means for promoting pharmaceutical products, particularly new drugs.

In the United States and in many other developed companies, pharmaceutical manufacturers are held to a high standard of quality and honesty in the production, marketing, and distribution of their products. Although sometimes viewed suspiciously by consumer groups and other observers, this industry has contributed to an unimpaired health status in this country.

The contributions of pharmaceutical research to our nation's health are enormous. Pharmaceutical discoveries have reduced morbidity and mortality in numerous areas including tuberculosis, coronary artery disease, arterial sclerosis, hypertension, and a whole host of infectious diseases. These products are in our everyday lexicon because they are so important to our health and well-being. We hear constantly about beta-blockers, angiotensin-converting enzyme (ACE) inhibitors, drugs for treating human immunodeficiency virus (HIV) infection, antibiotics, anti-inflammatories, and many, many other products.

The identification of the genetic origin of many diseases is now leading to clinical interventions and, in some instances, even curing an inborn genetic defect. Drug development is advancing so rapidly that products are becoming much more specific to the application, yielding therapies with far fewer side effects. Delivery mechanisms for drug therapies have also improved tremendously, with oral forms of many products that were previously delivered via intravenous transfusion now available and much more creative systems for drug delivery such as therapeutic patches for transdermal drug delivery.

The field of mental health services, as noted elsewhere, is a particular beneficiary of biomedical advances, with pharmacological agents now available for treating many illnesses (obsessive-compulsive disorder, anxiety disorder, depression, for example) that were previously difficult to control or cure. In other areas, recent pharmacological breakthroughs have led to improvement in treatments for metastatic breast cancer, human growth deficiency, rheumatory arthritis, stroke, lymphoma, hemophilia, organ rejection, and many other diseases. Many drugs have been, or are in the process of being, refined in their effectiveness, delivery efficiency, and safety profiles. In upcoming years creative progress will be achieved in treating various types of cancer, strokes, genetic errors, and in preventing both chronic and infectious disease.

REGULATION OF THE PHARMACEUTICAL INDUSTRY

As noted previously, the pharmaceutical industry is subject to extensive governmental regulation. Regulation is oriented primarily toward ensuring the quality of the product and the efficacy with which the product does what it says it does.

Regulation of this industry in the United States is primarily the responsibility of the U.S. Food and Drug Administration (FDA), which was established in 1938 by the U.S. Congress. The FDA is charged with the authority to ensure that pharmaceuticals and medical devices are relatively safe for use in human populations. The FDA also ensures that the marketing, production, and distribution of these products meet certain standards with regard to honesty and quality.

Pharmaceutical products and medical devices must be approved for sale by the FDA based on safety and effectiveness. In general, clinical studies must be performed that demonstrate that products are acceptably safe to use and they can be expected to achieve their stated goals.

The FDA establishes specific requirements that producers must meet to determine whether their products comply with federal regulation, thus allowing them to be sold in this country. Clinical studies demonstrating efficacy, safety, and effectiveness must be based on scientific, epidemiological principles.

In general, and for most drugs and products, the FDA requires a multipart demonstration of appropriateness prior to allowing a product to be marketed. To indicate that a new product is under development and will be considered for sale in the United States, a manufacturer must complete an Investigational New Drug (IND) application with the FDA. Clinical research is required to demonstrate safety and effectiveness of a drug.

Phase I clinical trials determine a drug's safety using a limited number of otherwise healthy subjects. In Phase II, a larger-scale test is performed, although the number of individual patients participating in Phase II is still limited. In the Phase II testing, the proposed new drug is actually tested on patients who are recognized with the medical condition that the drug is designed to treat. In Phase III, larger and longer clinical trials are performed using many more patients to assess more accurately the safety and efficacy of a drug. The remaining Phases IV and V follow drugs to determine more long-term effects, and to compare each proposed new drug with the already existing alternatives that are available in the marketplace.

The final approval for a new drug to be marketed in the United States is the New Drug Approval (NDA), which allows a manufacturer to market, distribute, and advertise a product. Although the time from initial research to new product marketing varies tremendously, in general the entire process can require anywhere from 5 to 7 years. In many instances, basic research may have been conducted for many years prior to the development of a specific new drug application. It has been estimated that as much as $200–800 million may be required to bring a new drug to market, starting with the initial basic research effort.

Drug research is time consuming and risky and many drug development efforts do not lead to a successful product in the marketplace. The regulatory review process itself is extremely complicated and requires a tremendous financial commitment. Recently, the FDA has worked to streamline and improve the effectiveness of the review process and to open accelerated reviews in certain situations. Nevertheless few drugs in early stage laboratory bench research will yield highly profitable products.

New drugs and many medical devices are patented to protect the intellectual property represented by the product. Patents ensure a significant payback period to reimburse the pharmaceutical company for the biomedical research and production and marketing investment required for a new product. Considerable controversy exists regarding drug industry regulation issues. These issues range from the extent to which the existing regulatory mechanisms ensure the safety and efficacy of a drug before it is brought to market to the appropriateness of the patent protection time interval prior to the availability of the product for copying by generic drug manufacturers.

Many drugs are developed for medical conditions that a relatively small number of people experience. Because a substantial cost is associated with bringing to market any new drug, and the market potential is somewhat limited for these drugs, Congress passed the Orphan Drug Act in 1983. This act allows modification of traditional approaches to new drug authorization and marketing to improve the economic advantages of developing drugs for limited markets. In addition, other special considerations are now provided for drugs aimed at terminal conditions and for the production of generic equivalent products.

The FDA is also responsible for the regulation of new medical devices. These include devices such as heart defibrillators, pacemakers, and surgical assist devices as well as a whole range of other medical devices needed for patient care. Again, there is considerable controversy about the role of the FDA in the regulation of medical devices, particularly with regards to possible inhibition of new creativity or creation of excess bureaucratic barriers to the introduction of technological advances.

ISSUES FACING THE PHARMACEUTICAL INDUSTRY IN THE FUTURE

The pharmaceutical and medical device industries face numerous challenges for the future. Individual for-profit pharmaceutical companies, in particular, face the challenge of maintaining an effective and long-lasting pipeline of new products. The substantial investment in biomedical research required to ensure future products requires immense capital and laboratory successes. Even given an effective biomedical research apparatus, pharmaceutical, biotechnology, and medical device companies must

still demonstrate the safety, effectiveness, and efficacy of their products prior to marketplace introduction. Once in the marketplace, these products must also continue to prove their worth from economic and clinical perspectives. This is a high-risk endeavor with substantial financial costs.

Increasingly, the pharmaceutical industry has been characterized by merger and consolidation activity. This trend is driven by the need to achieve economies of scale in the areas of biomedical research and marketing of products. The need to return profits to investors is particularly acute in light of recent stock price activity for most of these publicly held companies.

The pharmaceutical industry also faces political pressures related to product pricing. These pressures emanate from the increasing emphasis on drug therapies and their associated costs under insurance programs and national entitlement plans such as Medicare. Differential product pricing internationally results in further political pressure, since pharmaceutical prices tend to be highest in the United States, and similar drugs are substantially less expensive when purchased in many other countries. Patients who pay out of pocket for prescription products also react adversely to the high prices of patent-protected drugs. Rapid price increases and the significant premium assigned to new and innovative products further escalate the pricing issue.

Many ethical issues also face the pharmaceutical industry. These include the emphasis, particularly in the for-profit arena, on blockbuster products that are likely to yield the highest level of productivity and profitability at the expense of drugs aimed at more obscure medical conditions with a less likely payoff. Access to needed pharmaceuticals for individuals with little or no insurance or entitlement program availability is a further concern related to access to health care and issues of equity. There is a parallel international concern regarding the low level of availability of most modern pharmaceutical products in developing nations as well.

Managed care is introducing additional transformations into this industry. Many managed care plans, particularly those that are more stringent in their allocation of resources to pharmaceutical products, have established strict formularies under which more costly and newer prescription drug products are less likely to be utilized by their practitioners. Considerable effort is expended in many of these situations in determining the extent to which less expensive or older products can be safely utilized for patients instead of newer and more expensive pharmaceuticals. In addition, outright pressures attributable to reduced levels of reimbursement for prescription drugs and negotiated purchasing agreements have tended to enhance pricing pressures as well.

Governmental regulation of this industry is another area in which substantial uncertainty exists. In recent years, federal regulation of pharmaceuticals and medical devices has been improved through streamlined procedures and more rapid evaluation of new products by the government. However, the FDA is always facing trade-offs between accelerated reviews in decision making to facilitate new product introduction and the need to be somewhat cautious to ensure that drugs that are approved for marketing meet specific safety and efficacy standards. The United States is still more stringent in its review and approval processes than most other countries in the world. And the considerable costs associated with these review processes ultimately must be passed on to the consumer in the pricing of new products. An ongoing concern related to this issue is the need for continued surveillance and monitoring after products are introduced into the marketplace to ensure that if adverse consequences do subsequently present themselves, adequate regulatory response can be achieved. Again, the role of government remains an evolving and controversial issue for this industry.

Along these same lines, promising preliminary results have been achieved for the application of stem cell research for a variety of clinical situations. This technology, utilizing cells that can develop into a variety of clinical applications and other cutting edge developments in the pharmacological arena, pose complex ethical, political, economic, and medical issues and will require many years of development and evolution to achieve their eventual role in the health care system. Many issues also exist with regard to applied clinical research and the participation of patients in clinical studies, which are of immense importance in the development of new pharmacologic and other technological advances. Overall, technological diffusion of the spread of new technologies requires complex economic assessments as well as ongoing monitoring to determine the true payoff of various new technologies and the efficiencies with which they reach the patient care arena.

Ultimately, pharmaceuticals and medical devices are integral to our nation's health. Indeed, in recent years, biomedical advances suggest that pharmacologic agents will contribute more to the nation's health in the future in fighting disease than has ever been the case in the past. A thriving pharmaceutical industry, which has incentives to investigate and develop new products, is essential to the long-term viability of our own health. At the same time, important public policy issues must be addressed with regard to regulation, especially in the areas of safety, quality of product, and ongoing assurances of efficacy. As for many other areas of health care, concerns about cost must be weighed against issues of access and quality to assure that all Americans have the opportunity to take advantage of our increasing biomedical knowledge.

The pharmaceutical industry is a tremendous resource for the nation and an important contributor to the health of all Americans. Positioning this industry in a manner that rewards investors, protects consumers, and ensures the continuing proliferation of truly effective products will be a continuing challenge for the future of our nation.

TECHNOLOGICAL ADVANCES FOR HEALTH

Numerous other areas of biomedical and medical device progress have been evident over the past few decades. Among the many important areas of progress is imaging technology. Imaging had its origin with the development of X-ray machines. Today's imaging technologies, however, are vastly more sophisticated and provide a much greater range of clinical options for the diagnosis and monitoring of disease and illness. Imaging allows for the visualization of various internal organs and increasingly the assessment of their functional status. Using imaging technologies, less invasive approaches are available to the clinician to assess patient needs. Numerous imaging technologies are now available in clinical practice.

X-ray imaging has now been dramatically augmented by other techniques including ultrasound, which is increasingly widely used for a range of clinical applications; electron beam technology; positron emission technologies (PET), MRI, and a range of radiofrequency machines. Some of these technologies are also utilized for therapeutic intervention such as is the case for kidney stone treatment using electrolithotropters. Radiothermal and ultrasound technologies also are in use or are being developed for a range of treatment approaches to such diseases as cancer and many dermatological applications.

Imaging technologies are increasingly utilizing faster and more advanced computer systems for image analysis, display, and transmission. Computers themselves have an increased ability to identify areas of concern in images. Using the Internet and image transmission technologies, radiologists and other practitioners at remote sites can review the result of imaging procedures. The increasing use of faster scanning techniques, such as the electrobeam CT scanner, provides for comfortable and accurate imaging. A range of imaging technologies, including MRI and proton beam machines, are able to provide visualization of physiology, in addition to anatomy, such that functional status of organs and systems can be assessed. Most imaging technologies are now experiencing a dramatic expansion of sophistication, capabilities, application to clinical practice, and of course, in some instances, costs. The PET scan is another

example of a technology that provides information on function as well as structure. Enhanced imaging technologies are allowing for more effective and often less invasive surgical intervention.

Among the most important technological advances over the past quarter century has been the development of minimally invasive surgery. This class of surgical treatment allows for intervention with less patient disruption and discomfort. Minimally invasive surgery has been facilitated tremendously by the development of fiberoptic surgical equipment. Using this equipment, internal body parts can be visualized without performing open surgical procedures and associated equipment can be utilized to complete surgical interventions. Advancements in anesthesia have also greatly enhanced the ability to perform surgical procedures on an outpatient basis using minimally invasive technology. The health care delivery system has responded with the development of ambulatory surgery facilities, discussed elsewhere in this book. Examples of minimally invasive surgical procedures include arthroscopic, laparoscopic, and more recently cardiovascular procedures such as repair of structures in joints, aneurysms, the removal of gall bladders and other diseased body parts, and the use of angioplasty (often with stents) to repair cardiac blockages. Fine-needle aspiration of tumors is now utilized frequently for biopsies, replacing more invasive procedures. These technologies are constantly being improved and expanded, generally with excellent outcomes and high patient satisfaction.

One area in which these technologies have more recently been applied is in neurosurgery, using less invasive techniques to operate on the brain and related structures. Many other examples of the use of less invasive surgical procedures on the nervous system and on other parts of the body already exist in widespread clinical practice or are currently under development and will be available widely in the future. Patients benefit tremendously from less invasive procedures. For example, traditional cholecystectomy required a large abdominal incision and 3 to 5 nights of hospitalization followed by approximately 6 weeks of recovery. Laparoscopic cholecystrotomy requires a number of very small incisions and one night or less of hospitalization with only a few weeks of recovery. Parenthetically, the skill required of the surgeon is probably greater using less invasive technologies and total costs are probably about equal to the older techniques. Increasing use of these technologies combined with robots, computers, and three-dimensional imaging is part of today's revolution in higher quality, more effective, and more comfortable interventions for surgical needs.

The field of genetics is another huge area of biomedical progress. Now that the identification of the human genome has been completed, the next decade will witness a continuation of recent successes in identifying genetic defects associated with a wide range of diseases. Some diseases may be cured, some may be halted, and others may be controlled through intervention facilitated by the result of genetic research. Understanding the genetic foundations of a wide variety of diseases will likely lead to much more effective and specific interventions. Alzheimer's and other dementias, diabetes, cancer, heart disease, and many other types of disease categories will, at the least, be more effectively addressed with greater genetic understanding.

The genetic origins of many diseases are in the process of being identified. This in and of itself provides an exciting discovery of the origins of human illness. Genetic discoveries concerning mental illness are especially exciting with the identification of genes associated with susceptibility to a variety of diseases such as schizophrenia and severe depression.

Identification of genetic predispositions to various diseases raises complex concerns as well. If individuals can be profiled from a genetic prospective, should this information be available to potential employers and insurers, for example, or even potential spouses? The genetic revolution has many therapeutic advantages but also raises very difficult and complex social, ethical, and legal concerns.

Cloning is another area that raises many complicated moral issues.

Another important topic in biomedical research is vaccine development. Dating from the development of the smallpox vaccine by Edward Jenner in the 19th century, vaccination has been a major contributor to reductions in morbidity and mortality throughout the world. By preventing disease, vaccine products have the potential for tremendous contributions to health now and in the future. Many diseases, including smallpox, polio, measles, rubella, mumps, and diphtheria, have been eradicated completely or have been severely compromised in their impact as a result of these efforts.

Vaccine development has the potential to alleviate suffering from other diseases including acquired immunodeficiency syndrome (AIDS), some cancers, and some types of heart disease. In addition, enhanced vaccine development may provide greater protection for the population against the potential threat of terrorism from a biological event. Vaccine development using more sophisticated technologies, such as recombinant DNA, can address illness issues not previously thought to be susceptible to this type of intervention. Since we seem to be facing new infectious and chronic disease threats, terrorism, and other diseases such as severe acute respiratory syndrome (SARS) as a result of the increased mobility of the world's population, vaccine development should be a high priority for biomedical research.

Many other technological advances now and in the future will improve the quality and length of our lives. It is only through technology and the development of more efficient and effective delivery mechanisms that we can continue to achieve the principle goals of the nation's health care system. Our collective investment in technology including, pharmacological products, is essential to our well-being today and in the future.

Increasingly sophisticated computer systems are enhancing the ability of the scientist to conduct research. Computers and the Internet also facilitate the dissemination of information to health care professionals as well as to patients. Patient expectations are increasing as biomedical information becomes more available. An example of this situation is patient access to information on clinical studies. Biotechnology and pharmaceutical companies as well as the federal government are enhancing the availability of information about clinical studies for patient access and to facilitate enrollment of adequate numbers of patients in these studies. This represents an excellent example of Internet applications and the increasing role of consumers in participating in their own health care decision making. These issues also highlight the need to constantly evaluate new technologies along numerous parameters and to consider potential regulations of technological innovations. Such regulation is currently exemplified by the role of the FDA and by, in some states, the requirement for a certificate of need to add very expensive new technologies and facilities to existing organizations. The future role of regulation in technology and health care in general needs to be carefully assessed so as not to inhibit innovation but at the same time to ensure the appropriateness of technologies available to patients and the rapid diffusion of proven technologies to improve patient care. Evolving an adequate cadre of specially trained technical people to run all this new technology will also be an important issue for the future. The role of government as a payer, as exemplified by Medicare policy regarding paying for various clinical procedures as well as the Medicare drug benefit, further adds complexity to the overall analysis of these issues.

Other key issues in technology that are important include but certainly are not limited to the further development of electronic medical records to better organize patient information and improve access to care across multiple provider organizations. Electronic medical records have been under development for many years but now many of the larger health care organizations are finally implementing effective systems. Patient access to information using electronic medical records on the Internet and the protection of patient privacy will be important issues in the future. The use of telemedicine has been around for many years, particularly to support clinicians in rural areas. Telemedicine can be expected to expand with Internet applications such as remote control surgical equipment, remote reading of imaging tests, and transmission of patient clinical information. Finally, technology is increasingly playing a key role in the evaluation of the health care system and of individual provider performance such as physician report cards and insurer-required assessments of quality. Integrated information systems that combine patient information with evaluation standards and criteria will ultimately improve the management of the system and reduce such concerns as clinical areas. The promise of technology in the past has always delivered for the future and will continue to do so.

STUDY QUESTIONS

1. What is the nature of the pharmaceutical industry in the United States?
2. How is the success of the pharmaceutical industry related to the promotion of our nation's health?
3. How is the pharmaceutical industry in the United States regulated?
4. What are the primary trade-offs between the regulatory environment for pharmaceuticals and medical devices and public policy needs?

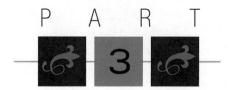

Paying for, Managing, Controlling, and Evaluating the System

This section discusses how we pay for and control the health care system. Issues concerning the evaluation of performance of the system are also discussed.

CHAPTER 11

Paying for Health Care

Chapter Objectives

1. To describe how individual providers are reimbursed in the health care system.
2. To describe how institutions are reimbursed in the health care system.
3. To identify major federal and state entitlement programs for the provision of health care services.
4. To examine the basic concepts of health insurance.
5. To explore alternative ways of paying for health services currently and in the future.

How we pay for health care has a tremendous effect on the behavior of providers, consumers, and institutions. The incentives that are created for each player by the payment mechanisms can change the way people behave.

This chapter discusses the general nature of the way health care is paid for and historical trends and current practices as they relate to both individual providers and institutions. Chapter 12 discusses the specific components of the managed care approach to organizing and paying for care, an approach increasingly prevalent in today's health care system.

Ideally, the ways in which we pay for health care should promote high-quality care, access to services for all Americans who need care, efficiency, and the provision of appropriate services to meet individual needs in the most cost effective way possible. Unfortunately, no single, ideal system exists for paying providers. The complexity and evolution of the nation's health care system have resulted in a plethora of payment approaches. These are discussed in this chapter in some detail.

PAYING INDIVIDUAL PROVIDERS

Individual professional providers, such as physicians and dentists, can be paid in a number of different ways. How providers are paid affects their behavior and the ways in which they marshal health care resources to benefit their patients. How providers are paid also affects how they interact with institutions, such as hospitals, and with government, employers, insurance companies, and the other players involved in the system.

Fundamental approaches to paying for individual professional services have remained fairly constant over time, although the specific nuances of each method have often been tweaked in one way or another. Since individuals respond to financial incentives, much of the effort in refining payment mechanisms has focused on creating incentives and, to a lesser extent, disincentives that are associated with various professional behavioral patterns. However, the difficulty of successfully incentivizing the provider, while at the same time containing costs and maximizing the quality of care for the consumer, has been and remains a tremendous challenge for the nation's health care system. In addition, in recent years some movement back to increased professional autonomy, especially for physicians, has occurred.

Professionals are generally paid in one of three ways or in a combination of two or more of these approaches. The general payment approaches are fee for service, capitation, and salary. Each of these approaches has a different set of incentives, and each affects physician-patient relationships, use of services, and quality of care in different ways.

Physician and other professional services reimbursement is a component of various health care plans and contractual arrangements. Under managed care programs, providers may be reimbursed through a variety of mechanisms, although each form of managed care typically utilizes specific elements of these primary reimbursement methodologies. Under managed care plans, furthermore, most providers are reimbursed based on contractual arrangements. These individual providers are termed participating providers and agree to accept the reimbursement mechanism specified in the contract for the managed care arrangement as discussed in more detail elsewhere. Medicare also utilizes the principle of participating physicians who agree to accept direct payment from the Medicare program for provider services. Under this program, by virtue of participating in a Medicare program, a provider agrees to a range of other practice constraints as they pertain to Medicare patients. Thus, reimbursement mechanisms for individual providers is complicated by virtue of the integration of these mechanisms with other constraints on the overall approach to reimbursement.

Fee-for-Service Reimbursement

The most traditional approach to professional services reimbursement is the fee-for-service mechanism. Fee for service is essentially piecework whereby professional providers, such as physicians or dentists, are paid a discrete fee for each specific service that is provided to a patient. How these fees are actually established can be complex, but the basic approach of fee-for-service payment is relatively clear cut.

Fee-for-service reimbursement assumes that services are provided in a set of discrete, defined, identifiable units that constitute the service itself. A service may be defined as an office visit or a procedure. A service may also be a comprehensive, or bundled, set of procedures, such as a vaginal delivery, for which one set fee might include the procedure and pre- and postoperative care.

The service unit is defined explicitly, although some vagueness may be introduced by assignment of the service unit. For example, an office visit might be a short or an intermediate visit.

Determination of payment for each discrete service under fee-for-service reimbursement has historically been based on what is termed usual, customary, and reasonable (UCR) fees. Essentially, UCR is a fee schedule for each physician listing discrete services provided by that physician and assigning a fee for each service. This fee is based on the physician's historical fee patterns and on the customary, or generally accepted, fee in the community for that service by that type of specialist.

Relative value scales are frequently used in fee-for-service reimbursement. These scales are used to weigh the time and complexity of each service and the relative weights between services. For example, a coronary artery bypass procedure might be the equivalent of five appendectomies. Medicare has used this methodology in changing reimbursement of physicians under the resource-based relative value (RBRV) scale system.

Numerous modifications of fee schedules are possible based on a great many factors, such as physician specialty and bundling of services. The central point is that an established, negotiated fee exists for each service provided.

Fee-for-service fee schedules can also be established without regard for the characteristics of the

provider, as is typical in indemnity insurance plans. Fee-for-service schedules can be highly arbitrary and, depending on the insurance plan, may or may not be subject to negotiation. Fee for service can be highly motivating and offers an opportunity, using carefully constructed fees to directly reimburse providers for specific services in an unambiguous manner.

The greatest problem with fee-for-service payment mechanisms is that they offer an incentive to provide many services and thus to increase the total amount of fees received. Particularly for unbundled services, physicians may be inclined to perform additional tests, visits, and procedures to increase their revenue under this approach. A provider's income is determined by the total number of services performed, the fees associated with each service, and the costs of running the practice.

To reduce the effect of pure fee for service, hybrid reimbursement schemes were developed that include certain features of both traditional indemnity and various forms of services mechanisms. These hybrid approaches include the combination of fee-for-service reimbursement with contractual agreements defining the level of reimbursement. Hybrid reimbursement mechanisms are typically found in some forms of managed care and protect the insurer against open-ended utilization and costs with additional protection provided for the consumer by limiting the extent to which providers can bill the patient beyond the reimbursable fee.

Capitation

A second mechanism for reimbursing professional services is capitation. Under capitation, a provider is paid a set fee, usually monthly, for each patient in his or her panel. A panel consists of the assigned patients, usually for primary care physicians, for whom the provider is responsible. Under capitation, the provider's set fee is not related to the volume of services delivered. Thus, regardless of the quantity of services required by a patient, the provider's reimbursement is the same monthly amount. As a result, capitation removes the incentive for increasing the volume of services to increase reimbursement levels. At the same time, however, a potential problem with capitation is that there may be underutilization of services, since there is no compensation for each service. Capitation is used by many managed care plans and by the British National Health Service.

Capitation rates can be adjusted for patient characteristics, such as age, to compensate a provider whose panel is likely to use more services. For any individual patient, once the capitation rate is set, most capitation payments are not adjusted for usage levels, except perhaps annually. An insurer may indemnify a provider against a patient with very high use resulting from serious illness. Capitation has many advocates owing to its disincentive for excessive utilization.

Conversely, capitation may lead to underutilization of services or the reluctance of providers to offer patients as much care as they may actually need. Under capitation, since the provider is paid the same amount regardless of the services offered to the patient, quality control and utilization review mechanisms are needed to ensure that patients still receive adequate care. These mechanisms may even include patient satisfaction surveys and other indicators of the consumer's perception of the care process.

Salaried Reimbursement

The third way in which professionals are reimbursed is salary. Under salary, which is used by government and some managed care organizations, a physician or other provider is paid a set monthly or annual salary. The salary itself is not dependent on the number of patients seen, the quantity of services provided, or the number of procedures performed.

Salaries are often adjusted for such factors as number of hours worked, physician specialty, length of employment experience, special capabilities, and administrative duties. A substantial portion of the nation's work force is paid a salary. However, among physicians, salary-based reimbursement has carried a stigma. While salary reimbursement removes the incentive for excessive utilization, productivity enhancement and monitoring measures may be necessary to ensure an adequate level of effort.

Various combinations of these three mechanisms are also possible. For example, it is very common for group practice physicians to be reimbursed with a salary plus an incentive compensation scheme tied to productivity based on revenue produced, patients seen, or services provided. These schemes attempt to combine the positive aspects of many reimbursement mechanisms to produce a productivity- and efficiency-enhancing end result.

Some insurance plans incorporate creative incentive programs. For example, some managed care programs, discussed in more detail in Chapter 12, have created risk-sharing reimbursement pools. Under these pools, physicians are paid based on fee-for-service reimbursement from a pool of funds, but with a bonus at the end of the year based on any funds remaining in the pool. The idea is to provide the productivity-enhancing benefits of fee for service with an incentive for cost containment. However, the success of these approaches has been mixed.

A difficult reimbursement problem is faced by group practice physicians when they see both managed care and fee-for-service patients. The incentives for these two categories of patients are diametrically opposed. Ultimately, of course, the objective of reimbursement methods should be to have all providers giving patients the most appropriate care, without under- or overproviding service, in a cost-effective and efficient manner.

INSTITUTIONAL REIMBURSEMENT

Institutions, particularly hospitals, have been reimbursed using a variety of schemes, none of which is ideal. The history of institutional reimbursement is also tied to federal Medicare and Medicaid program policies. Finding reimbursement mechanisms that offer the best mix of incentives for appropriate, efficient, but high-quality care has been difficult.

Hospitals were not historically paid in ways that promoted efficiency. Prior to October of 1983, Medicare reimbursed hospitals retrospectively, essentially paying whatever costs were incurred. The Medicare hospital reimbursement system computed an average per diem, or daily, cost for all Medicare patients in a facility. The hospital was reimbursed that per diem cost times the number of patient-days of care for Medicare patients.

The primary issue for negotiation between the hospital and Medicare was what costs would be included in the allowable cost computation. Medicare, for example, would not include the cost of neonatal intensive care services, since they ordinarily are not used by Medicare enrollees. Hospitals would try to include as much as possible in allowable costs. The hospital gift shop would not be included, while a pro rata share of administration, security, and other overhead services would be.

Under retrospective reimbursement then, any costs that could legitimately be included as Medicare-allowable costs were paid by the government. Hospitals with low occupancy or those which were inefficient were still paid based on their costs.

Other insurers paid hospitals in various ways. Many used some form of fee-for-service reimbursement, which, of course, does not provide a structure for cost containment or efficiency. Few payers have paid hospitals based on the "going rate" or "posted charges."

Hospital Prospective Payment

Recognizing the deficiencies of retrospective reimbursement, the U.S. Congress radically altered hospital reimbursement in October of 1983. The Congress mandated the use of prospective payment for most hospitals and hospital services after a phase-in period.

Under Medicare prospective payment, hospitals are reimbursed a set, preestablished fee for each patient admitted to the facility who is eligible for Medicare coverage. The set reimbursement is based on a categorization of possible diagnoses termed the diagnosis-related group (DRG). There are approximately 500 DRGs, or diagnostic categories. A patient who is admitted to the hospital is assigned a DRG that defines the amount of payment for that admission.

Except for unusual circumstances, called outliers, where there is specific justification for additional payment, the hospital receives one preestablished fee for all the services provided to the patient during that admission. If a patient requires more care, on average, than other patients for that diagnostic category, the hospital must make up the difference. Where patients require less care, the hospital retains the difference.

Since the DRG approach removes the incentive for additional use of resources by precluding any further payment by Medicare other than the single set fee, the hospital has a clear incentive to be efficient and cost conscious. In the prior system, retrospective reimbursement, there was no such incentive, since any additional services were fully reimbursed.

Under DRGs, there may be an incentive to discharge a patient too early or to underprovide services. Medicare attempts to monitor, through utilization review approaches, the care provided to patients to reduce the potential for underutilization. However, as with capitation and salary for professional services reimbursement, the potential for underutilization is very real.

Initially, prospective payment was quite profitable for many hospitals. However, in subsequent years, the government has reduced reimbursement levels in real dollar terms for most facilities, leading to increased financial pressures and much less potential for profitability from Medicare patients.

More recently, some hospitals and hospital systems have achieved greater profitability under Medicare reimbursement. However, in some instances, this profitability has yielded financial and legal liabilities, primarily as a result of action by the federal government. Hospitals have utilized mechanisms to increase reimbursement through perhaps questionable upcoding of admissions, or assigning a more expensive diagnosis than is appropriate, by taking advantage of provisions of the reimbursement laws that allow for extra payment for outliers or patients requiring unusual extra care, or other techniques that may or may not be considered allowable under the law. Unfortunately, since Medicare is a federal program, there are many opportunities to run afoul of federal laws, and in some instances the consequences for these actions can be tremendously costly in economic and personal terms.

Other payers, especially managed care plans, have negotiated discounts on their fees, further testing the financial viability of many hospitals. These trends are major factors in the problems faced in recent years by many of the national, for-profit hospital systems.

Under managed care, most plans, such as preferred provider organizations (PPOs) and health maintenance organizations (HMOs), reimburse hospitals on a negotiated and discounted per admission or on a fee-for-service basis. There is a range of specific arrangements for such reimbursement, most of which seek substantial discounts off the posted charges. More innovative arrangements, such as capitation, volume discounts, and bundling of services are also increasingly common.

The future of institutional reimbursement is likely to see a continuation of these recent trends. An increasingly competitive marketplace will dictate more discounting, more accountability, and greater expectations for cost containment. Institutions will have to become much more efficient, will have to affiliate with larger negotiating units, and will be expected to bundle together more services. High-quality care will be demanded by payers and consumers. Hospitals have not traditionally been at the forefront of cost containment and productivity enhancement, but they are now moving rapidly into these areas.

GOVERNMENT ENTITLEMENT PROGRAMS

Numerous government entitlement programs provide health services funding or direct provision of care. The federal government, the states, and local governments offer a variety of health-related programs targeted at selected populations. At the federal level, the largest programs are Medicare and Medicaid, the latter being a joint partnership with the states.

The Federal Medicare Program

Medicare is a national entitlement program that provides health care services funding, rather than actual services, to eligible individuals. In an entitlement program, eligibility is determined by the definitions contained in the relevant laws. For Medicare, services are generally provided to individuals who are U.S. citizens or permanent residents and who have attained the age of 65. People on permanent Social Security disability are also eligible for Medicare coverage regardless of their age. While the specific details of the Medicare program are rather complex, the basic thrust of the program is to facilitate older Americans' access to medical care. The program was enacted into law during President Lyndon B. Johnson's Great Society in the mid-1960s.

Medicare covers most somatic acute care services but has limited coverage for mental health and long-term care. Individuals eligible for Medicare coverage can obtain benefits under two types of programs. Medicare is paid for from employer and employee contributions for part A, the hospital program discussed later in this chapter, and by monthly beneficiary premiums, general tax revenue, interest, and other sources for Medicare's part B, the primarily physician and outpatient services part discussed in more detail later also.

The Medicare indemnity program is the traditional form. In this part of the Medicare program, enrollees seek services in the community from their

Table 11.1. Medicare Provisions (Summary)

Medicare is a health insurance program for:

- People age 65 or older.
- People under age 65 with certain disabilities.
- People with end-stage renal disease (permanent kidney failure requiring dialysis or a kidney transplant).

Medicare part A

Medicare part A (hospital insurance) covers inpatient care in hospitals, critical access hospitals, and skilled nursing facilities (not custodial or long-term care). It also helps cover hospice care and some home health care.

Cost: Most people do not have to pay a monthly premium for part A because they or a spouse paid Medicare taxes while he or she was working.

Medicare part A covers medically necessary:

Hospital stays: Semiprivate room, meals, general nursing, and other hospital services and supplies. Inpatient mental health care in a psychiatric facility is limited to 190 days in a lifetime.

Skilled nursing facility care: Semiprivate room, meals, skilled nursing and rehabilitative services, and other services and supplies (after a related 3-day inpatient hospital stay).

Home health care: Part-time or intermittent skilled nursing care and home health aide services, physical therapy, occupational therapy, speech-language therapy, medical social services, durable medical equipment (such as wheelchairs, hospital beds, oxygen, and walkers), medical supplies, and other services.

Hospice care: For people with a terminal illness; includes drugs for symptom control and pain relief, medical and support services from a Medicare-approved hospice, and other services not otherwise covered by Medicare.

Medicare part B

Medicare part B (medical insurance) covers doctors' services and outpatient hospital care. It also covers some other medical services that part A does not cover, such as some of the services of physical and occupational therapists, and some home health care.

Cost: The Medicare part B premium each month was $66.60 in 2004.

Medicare part B covers medically necessary:

Medical and other services: Doctors' services (not routine physical exams), outpatient medical and surgical services and supplies, diagnostic tests, ambulatory surgery center facility fees for approved procedures, and durable medical equipment (such as wheelchairs, hospital beds, oxygen, and walkers). Also covers second surgical opinions, outpatient mental health care, and outpatient occupational and physical therapy including speech-language therapy. (These services are also covered for long-term nursing home residents.)

Clinical laboratory services: Blood tests, urinalysis, some screening tests, and more.

Home health care: Part-time or intermittent skilled nursing care and home health aide services, physical therapy, occupational therapy, speech-language therapy, medical social services, durable medical equipment (such as wheelchairs, hospital beds, oxygen, and walkers, medical supplies, and other services).

Outpatient hospital services: Hospital services and supplies received as an outpatient as part of a doctor's care.

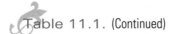 Table 11.1. (Continued)

Medicare also may cover:

- Ambulance services.
- Artificial eyes, artificial limbs that are prosthetic devices, and their replacement parts.
- Braces.
- Chiropractic services (limited), for manipulation of the spine to correct a subluxation.
- Emergency care.
- Eyeglasses after cataract surgery with an intraocular lens.
- Foot exams for diabetes-related nerve damage.
- Hearing and balance exams if ordered by your doctor to see if medical treatment is needed.
- Oral immunosuppressive drug therapy for transplant patients.
- Kidney dialysis.
- Medical supplies such as ostomy bags, surgical dressings, splints, casts, and some diabetic supplies.
- Limited preventive services.
- Prosthetic/orthotic devices, including breast prosthesis after mastectomy.
- Transplants—heart, lung, kidney, pancreas, intestine, bone marrow, cornea, and liver (under certain conditions and in Medicare-certified facilities only).
- X-rays, MRIs, CT scans, EKGs, and some other diagnostic tests.

usual sources of care. Claims are submitted on their behalf to fiscal intermediaries, who process the claims under contract to the Medicare program's administrative unit within the Department of Health and Human Services.

The principal components of the Federal Medicare Program for the indemnity option are parts A and B. Part A generally incorporates benefits pertaining to inpatient hospital services while part B is the program component that funds professional and other noninstitutional services. Funding for part A services is primarily provided from federal sources, while part B requires a larger enrollee contribution. Medicare also provides coverage to eligible Americans with end-stage renal disease under a specific part of the program's legislation. Enrollees are eligible for hospice care in the event of a terminal illness. Individuals who are currently working and are eligible for employer-sponsored health care benefits through their source of employment may utilize Medicare indemnity program coverage only as a secondary benefit program

to supplement their employer's plan. The shift of responsibility for these individuals and their spouses in the 1980s as a result of congressional legislative action has significantly reduced potential federal liability. However, with the aging of the population, and increasing costs for health care, many employers are reducing the scope of coverage or are eliminating completely coverage for retirees and their spouses, putting the burden for these individuals, once they reach the age of Medicare eligibility, back on the federal government and on individuals themselves.

A summary of the traditional indemnity Medicare program is presented in Table 11.1. A summary of enrollee costs is presented in Table 11.2. An alternative to the traditional Medicare indemnity program using managed care plans is presented in Table 11.3.

The 2003 Medicare Legislation signed into law by President George W. Bush contains further revisions and refinements of the Medicare program intended to be phased in over a significant number

Table 11.2. Medicare Enrollee Costs (in 2003)

Medicare, part A enrollee costs

Hospital stays for each benefit period:

- A total of $840 for a hospital stay of 1–60 days.
- $210 per day for days 61–90 of a hospital stay.
- $420 per day for days 91–150 of a hospital stay.
- All costs for each day beyond 150 days.

Skilled nursing facility care for each benefit period:

- Nothing for the first 20 days.
- Up to $105 per day for days 21–100.
- All costs beyond the 100th day in the benefit period.

Home health care:

- Nothing for home health care services.
- 20% of the Medicare-approved amount for durable medical equipment.

Hospice care:

A copayment of up to $5 for outpatient prescription drugs and 5% of the Medicare-approved amount for inpatient respite care (short-term care given to a hospice patient so that the usual caregiver can rest). Medicare generally does not pay for room and board except in certain cases. For example, room and board are not covered for general hospice services while a patient is a resident of a nursing home or a hospice's residential facility. However, room and board are covered for inpatient respite care and during short-term hospital stays.

Medicare, part B enrollee costs

Medical and other services each year:

- $100 deductible (once per calendar year).
- 20% of Medicare-approved amount after the deductible.
- 20% for all outpatient physical, occupational, and speech-language therapy services. (No coverage limit for these therapy services provided by a hospital outpatient facility. If provided at another type of outpatient setting, $1,590 coverage limit per year for occupational therapy services, and $1,590 limit per year for physical and speech-language therapy services combined).
- 50% for outpatient mental health care.

Clinical laboratory services:

No enrollee payments for Medicare-approved services.

Home health care:

- Nothing for Medicare-approved services.
- 20% of the Medicare-approved amount for durable medical equipment.

Outpatient hospital services:

A coinsurance or copayment amount, which may vary according to the service.

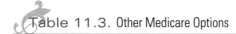

Table 11.3. Other Medicare Options

Medicare + Choice Plans

Coverage through the original Medicare plan or Medicare + Choice plan is available

- Medicare managed care plans:
  Enrollee can go only to doctors, specialists, or hospitals on the plan's list. May have to choose a primary care doctor and get referrals to see a specialist.
- Medicare private fee-for-service plans:
  Enrollee can go to any doctor or hospital that accepts the terms of the plan's payment. The private company, rather than the Medicare program, decides how much it will pay and what the enrollee pays for services.
- Medicare preferred provider organization plans (PPOs):
  In most of these plans, enrollees use doctors, specialists, and hospitals on the plan's list (network). Enrollee can go to doctors, specialists, or hospitals not on the plan's list, but it may cost extra. Enrollees do not need referrals to see specialists.
- Medicare specialty plans:
  these plans provide more focused health care for some people. You join one of these plans, you get all your Medicare health care to manage a specific disease or condition.

Medigap Policies

A Medigap policy is a health insurance policy sold by private insurance companies to fill the "gaps" in original Medicare plan coverage. There are 10 standardized Medigap plans called "A" through "J". The front of a Medigap policy must clearly identify it as "Medicare Supplement Insurance." Each plan A through J has a different set of benefits. Plan A covers only the basic (core) benefits. These basic benefits are included in all the plans A through J. Plan J offers the most benefits. Enrollees pay a premium to the insurance company.

---

of years. These provisions include a broader array of privately offered health care plans and benefits to be made available through the Medicare program and a partial outpatient prescription package. The legislation increases the complexity of the Medicare program and does not fundamentally address the need to consider redesigning the program and simplifying the provisions under which services are offered to enrollees. However, further evolution of the Medicare program will likely clarify many of these important issues.

Medicare benefits are established uniformly across the country based on the actions of the U.S. Congress. The program can be changed through legislative action. For example, the method of reimbursement of hospitals under the traditional Medicare program was changed in 1983 by the Congress in an effort to reduce increases in costs by changing the structure of hospital reimbursement.

Another interesting illustration of the political environment for the Medicare program is the initiative in 1988 to enact a catastrophic coverage plan under Medicare to provide protection against the most serious situations that an enrollee could face, exclusive of expanded coverage for long-term care. Although the legislation was initially passed, it was subsequently repealed as a result of political pressure from organized groups purporting to represent Medicare enrollees because of concerns by these groups that the catastrophic coverage was associated with substantial additional enrollee premium costs and potential additional taxation.

Medicare is funded by the federal government and enrollees but covers only approximately half of all health care costs for enrollees. The remaining costs are paid for by individuals themselves, by other entitlement programs, usually Medicaid, or by supplemental insurance from private companies sold to augment Medicare coverage. Supplemental plans must now meet specific federal guidelines and are offered in a variety of options which allow individuals to select how much additional coverage they wish to purchase.

The Medicare program has generally been successful in increasing access to care for older Americans. As a major purchaser of services, and particularly of hospital care, Medicare has had tremendous impact on the nation's health care delivery system. In spite of its limitations, the program has been fairly well run and has generally met with a high degree of consumer acceptance.

A second option for Medicare enrollees is to elect a Medicare HMO. Medicare contracts with community-based HMOs and other managed care providers to enroll Medicare eligibles in these plans. Individuals who elect this option forgo their traditional Medicare indemnity benefits. They then obtain care from a managed care organization, similar to an employee's use of company-provided benefits.

Over the past few years, the Medicare program has also initiated expanded efforts to control fraud and abuse among providers. These efforts include much more stringent regulations that providers must adhere to, which relate to such matters as self-dealing and outright fraud, inflated billing, and conflicts of interest. Medicare's Peer Review Organizations serve as a watchdog over the provision of services by reviewing provider claims and other information to detect fraud.

The Medicare program had not been fundamentally changed since its inception until recent congressional action. Except for the addition of managed care program options (Medicare Advantage), coverage of patients with end-stage renal disease, and some changes in institutional and professional services reimbursement, the Medicare program is not that different from its early conception 40 years ago. At the same time, health care delivery, medical technology, and the institutions and providers that constitute the system have all changed radically.

Over time Medicare has increased its reimbursement options recognizing these changes such as cov-erage for ambulatory surgery and home health services. However, many believe that the program should be fundamentally revised with significant changes that recognize the new biomedical world that we live in today. Among the most prominent areas in need of change, of course, has been a prescription drug benefit for outpatient services, not initially included in the Medicare program. With biomedical research increasingly focused on the development of outpatient pharmacological therapies such a change would seem to be a natural development. Political and economic considerations have long thwarted such an update to the Medicare program. Recent changes are dramatic illustrations of the intensity of the debate and the conflicting political perspectives. The Medicare program has been held hostage to national political and economic concerns and as a creation of the Congress, implementing change and major program updates will likely always continue to be a highly politicized issue.

MEDICAID

The Medicaid program, unlike Medicare, is a welfare or transfer program and a joint effort on the part of the federal government and the states. Medicaid is targeted at medically indigent individuals. It is a financing mechanism designed to facilitate access to community-based health care for people who otherwise have limited financial access.

The Medicaid program is jointly funded by the federal government and the states. In contrast to the Medicare program, for which benefits and eligibility are specified uniformly across the nation, the Medicaid program varies from state to state. Each state has some prerogatives in specifying benefits and eligibility.

The federal Medicaid program was enacted in July of 1965 as Title XVI of the Social Security Act. Combined with the federal Medicare program, these legislative initiatives represented tremendous enhancement of the safety net for older and low-income Americans. Prior to this point in time, individuals received care through charity hospital services and services donated by physicians and other providers or paid under sliding scale schemes that adjusted fees for income.

The Medicaid program, formerly a federal-state cooperative effort, funded approximately 50 percent by each, is administered separately by each state, under broad federal guidelines. Medicaid eligibility is targeted toward low-income individuals and families in a variety of categories including certain groups of the aged, the blind and disabled, low-income and medically needy adults and children, and selected other categories of eligibility.

Because the program is designed to provide services on a temporary rather than permanent basis, as compared to the Medicare program, eligibility for services is reevaluated for individuals periodically under welfare programs such as the Temporary Assistance and Needy Families and Supplemental Security Income programs. Certain pregnant and postpartum women, as well as disabled and other individuals whose incomes are within certain low-income parameters are also eligible. Low-income, medically needy, aged individuals, although representing a relatively small proportion of total beneficiaries, also represent a high percentage of total expenditures owing to the high cost of long-term care and nursing home services. States have a certain degree of flexibility in the determination of which benefits they will provide, which population groups will be eligible, and in the specific arrangement of services. Since the states themselves administer these programs, under federal guidelines, there are many differences across the nation in state Medicaid programs.

All state Medicaid programs generally provide hospital inpatient and outpatient services; physician and other professional services; nursing home and certain related, medically necessary, long-term care services; some nurse-provided services; some educational programs; screening services; and to a varying degree, dental care. Optional services under federal guidelines may extend the minimum required services to include a wider array of clinical care, drugs, eye care, enhanced dental care, and certain other services.

Since state Medicaid programs are administered differently state by state, there are many different examples of program operations. Increasingly, forms of managed care have been introduced into state Medicaid programs as an effort to improve operations, enhance continuity of care, and contain the growth and the cost of the program by shifting utilization and cost risks to provider organizations and to individuals.

State Medicaid programs in most instances do not pay providers particularly well. Reimbursement levels are generally below those of the Medicare program and are often extremely low by community standards. Individuals eligible for both Medicare and Medicaid, termed the Medi/Medi population, have their care generally administered by the Medicaid programs. Medicaid recipients may be required to pay nominal portions of their care charges. Arizona is the only state that does not participate in the traditional Medicaid program, having opted out to provide these services through a unique effort of its own design, ultimately in an effort to reduce state costs.

Many other entitlement programs for specific population needs have been developed by government. These include, but are certainly not limited to, the Veterans Administration health care system; various programs targeted to women, infants, and children; and a federal program aimed at facilitating financial access to kidney dialysis (End Stage Renal Disease program), which is administered under the Medicare program.

Other programs have provided funds to subsidize services directly or to develop health care resources. Still, an estimated 9 to 40 million Americans have no coverage at any point in time. These efforts include various somatic and mental health community clinics and local government clinics targeted to such needs as venereal disease control.

Still facing the quandary of how to provide services to many medically indigent individuals while containing costs, most state Medicaid programs are continuing to experiment with alternative approaches. These include various forms of managed care and risk sharing, contracting for services, and applying other patient management techniques, often under federal waivers that allow for experimentation that may improve the quality and quantity of care.

Further complicating the situation after the late 1990s boom was the recession and continuing sluggish economy, which resulted in relatively high unemployment, underemployment, and an inherent drag on health care benefits and affordability. Combined with an increasing shift of costs to employees and other consumers, Medicaid and other social programs have seen their caseload and care level obligations increase. Cutbacks in coverage and beneficiary eligibility have, on the one hand, moderated the fiscal impact for certain programs, but have also increased the demands on the local government safety nets as individuals increasingly fall between the cracks.

The business cycle can be particularly harsh on these types of programs because downturns increase the number of individuals potentially eligible for coverage as a result of economic circumstances, but also lower government receipts as a result of erosion in the tax base and in economic activity overall. The economic and political pressures on politicians and on government, particularly at the local level, are quite intense as a result of these circumstances. Ultimately, only an economic expansion combined with an improvement in local, state, and federal government finances can help to alleviate these burdens. The need to develop more permanent solutions to providing care and coverage for those in greatest need continues regardless of the economic cycle, and these issues must eventually be addressed with an eye toward longer term and more permanent solutions.

COMMERCIAL INSURANCE

Private insurance companies such as Aetna and Travelers originally entered the health insurance market to provide a full range of insurance products to their customers. Indeed, the insurance industry traditionally did not focus on health care products.

Health insurance in this country had its origins in the nonprofit sector through the initiative of provider organizations. Further back in history, health insurance can be traced to mutual benefit societies in Europe during the 1800s, which attempted to provide relief for industrially employed low-income individuals. Commercial health insurance should also be differentiated from government programs to protect populations at risk. The former is often termed voluntary health insurance while the latter is often called social health insurance.

Today, the vast majority of employed Americans have some form of voluntary or private health insurance or are eligible for coverage under a federal entitlement program. However, for all population groups under all of these programs, significant limits in the scope of coverage exist and many expenses have to be borne by the consumer. Individuals losing employment, or those working for employers without employer-sponsored health care benefits, face significant challenges, as do many persons who fall between the cracks such as early retirees not yet eligible for Medicare without employer-sponsored health care benefits. Since many individuals and dependents receive health care benefits as a result of employment, divorce and other social circumstances can adversely affect health care coverage. Some circumstances such as loss of employment due to illness can be particularly challenging. Even with federally mandated options for continuing postcoverage employment, the challenges are substantial since such coverage must be paid for by the enrollee and is available for only a limited time.

There are a number of other important related programs. Worker's compensation programs are required of employers in all 50 states but vary tremendously in their design and operation. These programs are intended to provide protection for workers injured as a result of employment. Costs for worker's compensation insurance and other mandated benefits are figured into the pricing of all goods and services sold in the United States and are never a "freebee".

Local government is the provider of last resort. Individuals who do not have access to health insurance or are not eligible for a government entitlement program must also be provided health care services when in need. Local governments organize and operate or arrange for and pay for welfare type services for physical and mental health problems for this population. Ultimately, one way or another, all Americans receive some degree of health care services, at least in the most serious situations, but these arrangements are unlikely to be ideal or effective in many instances.

Health insurance had its modern origins in the United States during World War II. Wage and price controls during the war limited what employers could offer their employees and what unions could seek to benefit their members. Health insurance was seen as a desirable expansion of employer benefits. Unions could argue that the acquisition of health insurance benefits was extremely valuable for their membership, and employers could point to this benefit as a tangible and meaningful, almost thoughtful, alternative to wages for employees.

To further sweeten the pot, health care benefits are tax deductible for the employer and tax free for the employee. Thus employees need not pay taxes on the value of this benefit. If employees had to buy these benefits with after-tax dollars, the real cost to them would be much greater.

The extent to which the cost to employers of health care benefits has reduced wages is unknown. Consideration has been given in recent years to taxing health care benefits that exceed a certain level.

The early development of health insurance benefits was undertaken by nonprofit Blue Cross and Blue Shield plans. Blue Cross was started when the hospital industry wanted a mechanism to spread the risk of hospitalization costs among members of the community to ensure that hospitals would be reimbursed for those expenses. Physicians, seeing the benefits of such insurance coverage, jumped on the bandwagon with the establishment of Blue Shield plans.

Health care insurance initially was focused on inpatient hospital care and eventually spread to other benefit categories, particularly physician services, drugs, and ancillary services. Much more recently, dental services and other areas of health care have been increasingly covered as well.

The growth of voluntary, for-profit health insurance plans is more recent, evolving, as mentioned previously, from the need for these companies to offer a full range of products to their clientele. Health insurance has not always been profitable for private health insurers. A competitive marketplace and restrictions on reimbursement under entitlement programs led to financial problems for many Blue Cross and Blue Shield plans and pressures on profits for the for-profit companies. Some hospital management companies have also ventured into the health insurance arena, generally not very successfully.

With the expansion of managed care and movements toward health care reform, the industry has shifted its focus toward prepaid plans. Some insurance companies have purchased medical groups or have affiliated with health care systems to have more direct control over their provider networks. Other insurers have used contractual arrangements with community providers to put together managed care plans. Some health care systems have themselves developed insurance products, bypassing the traditional third parties.

Consolidation in the Industry

Over the last decade, there has been tremendous consolidation of health care plans, programs, and providers, with the creation of ever-larger networks insuring or providing services. Particularly in the Northeast and Midwest and on the West Coast, this trend toward consolidation has led to battles of the Goliaths, with large, integrated systems battling one another in the marketplace.

At the same time as the insurance industry and the provider systems have been forming alliances and developing their competitive strategies through integrated networks, many employers have sought to bypass the insurance industry entirely. Self-funded employer plans have been developed. Employers are either contracting directly with large, multispecialty group practices and health systems or working through administrative organizations, such as third-party administrators (TPAs). These organizations put together and manage health care systems, perform claims and utilization review, and provide oversight for employers on a contractual basis. Employers may buy reinsurance that protects them against any unusually high claims.

An extensive reorganization of the health insurance industry has occurred over the last 10 years. Some traditional multiline insurance companies have sold their health care businesses to other corporations while a number of large insurance companies have focused on health care, as in the case of Aetna. Increasing specialization and the development of a range of products have led to competitive marketplaces in many communities between formerly traditional insurance companies, various iterations of the traditional Blues, and a variety of large managed care only companies such as Kaiser. Employers and providers face increasingly intense negotiations with these large insurance entities.

Tremendous cost pressures brought on in part by new technology and by many other factors including inflation and aging of the population have led to premium increases and cost shifting to employees through higher copayments. Even relatively comprehensive employer-sponsored health insurance plans today are associated with significant financial responsibility on the consumer's part. Retirees who are covered under employer-sponsored health plans but who are not yet eligible for Medicare have been particularly hard hit by cost increases and by the outright termination of employer-sponsored coverage.

The proliferation of health insurance plans and programs, of providers, and of organizational forms has resulted in tremendous diversity across the country. Managed care, in particular, has grown greatly in some areas of the country, while other areas cling to more traditional forms of reimbursement. The increasing consolidation of the industry

and some decline in the viability of weaker players among insurers and providers is rapidly changing the face of the industry. As the nation moves toward fewer, but larger and more integrated, provider and insurance arrangements, issues of maintaining a competitive marketplace, of antitrust, and of quality of care become much more important.

THE PRINCIPLES OF HEALTH INSURANCE

Insurance is designed to spread risk among a large number of people. Insurance protects against unwanted, unexpected, and undesirable events. Life insurance is a typical example of an insurance product ideally suited to spreading the risk among a large number of people. The likelihood of an adverse consequence for any individual can be determined using life tables. Each individual in the risk pool is protected against an unexpected and unwanted event, while the cost of protecting the entire pool of people is predictable.

Health insurance is designed to protect against undesirable, unwanted, and unpredictable events over a time period. When individuals seek insurance knowing that they already have a problem, then the insurer is not really protecting against an undesirable or unwanted event. To protect against these situations, insurers screen potential enrollees for the risk of adverse selection. In health care, screening may involve taking a history or conducting a physical examination.

Health insurance does not fit the traditional concepts of insurance. Many aspects of health insurance are not wanted or undesirable and are, in fact, the result of initiatives by the patient or the provider. The risk experience of even a large group of individuals is often difficult to predict accurately. Utilization is heavily influenced by many factors, such as the way services are organized and incentive compensation arrangements. Providers themselves generate much demand for care, a somewhat unique attribute of the health care industry.

Health insurance coverage varies tremendously throughout the population. The level of coverage, patient responsibility for payment, and the exact services that are covered, even under entitlement programs, differ by geographic location or even among employee groups. Minimum benefits exist primarily when regulated for certain HMOs, entitlement programs, and state-regulated insurance plans and for state or federally mandated benefits.

Mechanisms of Insurance

This part of the chapter discusses some of the mechanisms by which health insurance operates. Particular attention is directed toward the terminology used in the health insurance field.

Health insurance is a contractual arrangement between the insured and the insurer. Sometimes health insurance also involves contracts between the insurer and the providers, especially under managed care. All aspects of the insurance coverage are defined by the contract. As an enrollee in a health insurance plan, you should be cognizant of every provision of the contract as summarized in the plan summary of benefits.

Health insurance plans and entitlement programs are offered to individuals who meet specific criteria. These people are deemed to be eligible (the eligibles) for the coverage. Eligibility under entitlement programs, such as Medicare and Medicaid, is determined by government policy and may include such factors as age and income. Eligibility under an employer-sponsored plan is usually determined by employment status, such as whether an individual is working the qualifying minimum number of hours per week, or other provisions of the employment contract.

Group plans are offered under master contracts to employees and, in some instances, to other types of groups. Some nonhealth insurance products, for example, accident coverage, may be offered through affinity groups, such as membership organizations. Health insurance ·is offered primarily through employer groups.

In addition to group plans, insurance companies also offer individual plans marketed directly to unaffiliated consumers. Under these plans, an individual not associated with a group applies for coverage and is evaluated by the insurer to determine eligibility. Insurers use underwriting criteria developed by their actuaries to assess insurability.

Insurance companies are concerned about adverse risk selection when they market individual plans. Insurance is primarily a means of spreading risk for undesirable events across large groups. In group plans, the possible effect of adverse risk selection is contained by signing up large numbers of employees and many groups. In individual plans, where anyone can walk through the door and apply for coverage, adverse risk can easily occur.

A related concept is moral hazard, the risk that an individual will change his behavior if he knows that he is covered by an insurance policy, perhaps, for example, paying less attention to healthy behaviors since subsequent illness would be covered by health insurance.

To protect against adverse risk selection under individual plans, insurance companies will, for example, exclude anyone with a history of cancer or serious cardiovascular disease. In group plans, risk is spread across many more people, and the premium is based on the employee group's total previous experience, which is termed experience rating.

Individuals who are covered by a health insurance plan, including in managed care or entitlement programs, are termed enrollees. Enrollees receive benefits under an insurance plan. Benefits are those services that are covered as specified in the contract. Historically, health insurance has had greatest coverage of in-hospital, ancillary, and, more recently, ambulatory care services. The shift of care and coverage to the outpatient or ambulatory side has been an important trend over the past 30 years.

Benefits can be restricted to protect the insurance company against excessive utilization or other risks. Exclusions are situations or services that are not covered at all in the benefits. Typical exclusions include preexisting conditions, terrorism, acts of war, acts of God, plastic and reconstructive surgery performed for purely cosmetic reasons, experimental medical procedures and therapies, and services not provided by a licensed physician. Pregnancy and delivery have at times also been excluded. Most medical insurance plans do not cover dental care and certain other conditions of the mouth.

In addition to exclusions, insurance companies can protect themselves by limiting benefits. Limitations may be expressed in dollars or in numbers of services. For example, mental health benefits are often limited to a predefined number of visits per year. Dollar limitations include maximum annual or lifetime coverage under a plan, typically one million dollars or more. All of these conditions on coverage are legitimate and legal unless there are governmentally mandated coverages. These conditions are, of course, defined by the terms of the insurance contract.

The fee that the enrollee pays for insurance coverage is the premium. This may be paid by an individual directly or by an employer on behalf of the employee. All or a portion of an employee's contribution to the premium may be deducted from his or her paycheck. Premiums are usually remitted monthly or quarterly.

Health insurance plans are generally limited to coverage for somatic and certain mental health conditions. Other plans typically cover dental, vision, and occasionally prescription drug benefits, although this last category is frequently incorporated into a health care medical coverage plan.

Dental plans are available in both traditional indemnity format as well as in managed care alternatives. Dental insurance typically available through group coverage as an additional employer-sponsored or employee benefit covers specific services related to preventive care, restorative services, oral surgery, endodontics, and perodontics. Dental plans typically include deductibles and coinsurance although preventive services are often covered without a copayment for a specified number of services per year as an incentive to improve oral health.

Copayments for many other services are typically as high as 50 percent. Dental plans often have total annual allowable coverages and may also have lifetime maximum coverages for such services as orthodonture. Dental plans augment medical plans that do not cover most of these services. Managed care, particularly HMO dental plans, require conformance to strict delivery arrangements with services provided by capitated dentists. Dental PPOs have somewhat greater flexibility for patients and typically have higher total out-of-pocket costs, particularly when patients seek care outside of the contracted provider network.

Vision plans, like dental plans, serve as an additional benefit in employer-sponsored programs. Vision plans usually provide some coverage for routine eye exams and eyeglasses and contact lenses. These plans are not primarily for the treatment of medical diseases of the eye, but rather are focused on vision correction and prophylaxis. The level of coverage and consumer costs vary greatly.

Service Versus Indemnity Insurance

There are two primary contractual approaches to health insurance. In indemnity arrangements, the insurance company has a contract with the customers who are the covered beneficiaries or, in insurance parlance, the covered lives. Indemnity insurance does not involve any relationship between the insurance company and the providers.

In indemnity insurance, when an individual incurs a loss, such as a hospitalization, the insurance company agrees to pay the beneficiary a set dollar fee. Thus, the insurance contract covers a risk, and when there is a loss, pays a set fee for that event. In other forms of insurance, such as casualty or life, a parallel mechanism exists to compensate someone who experiences a loss; a set, predetermined amount is paid to the beneficiary of the policy.

Indemnity reimbursement to the beneficiary is often not based on the fee charged to the consumer by the provider. As a result, providers may charge fees in excess of what the insurance pays for such losses. The consumer is usually responsible for paying the excess fee. As a result, indemnity insurance holds significant financial risk for the insured. Figure 11.1 illustrates the relationships that exist in indemnity insurance.

A second form of insurance, typified by many early Blue Shield plans, is service insurance. Under service insurance, the insurance company agrees to provide services rather than dollars to the insured. To provide service, the insurance company contracts with local providers in the community, such as hospitals and physicians. The early service plans were the precursors of many of today's managed care plans.

In service plans, there are contractual relationships between the insurance company and the providers, in addition to relationships with the consumer. These relationships are illustrated in Figure 11.1.

The provider who participates in service plans agrees to an established fee schedule and further agrees not to charge the enrollee in excess of the allowable or agreed-upon fee. These conditions are enforced by formal, contractual relationships. As a result, in service plans, consumers generally must use providers who have contractual relationships with the

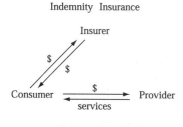

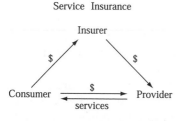

Figure 11.1. Insurance Contractual Relationships

plan. In return, the consumer receives protection against fees that exceed the approved, negotiated rate.

In indemnity plans, consumers can seek care from any provider of their choice, since no contract is required between insurers and providers. In a service plan, since contractual relationships must exist in order for there to be agreed-upon reimbursement, consumers must use providers who contract with the plan.

More Health Care Terms

Most insurance arrangements require patients to pay part of their cost of care. Those services for which there are no benefits, such as cosmetic plastic surgery or over-the-counter drugs, may also be termed uncovered services. Patient payments for uncovered services are paid out of pocket, meaning out of the patient's pocket, as mentioned previously. Out-of-pocket health care costs constitute a surprisingly large fraction of all health care expenditures, particularly with the lack of coverage for long-term care and requirements for patients to pay part of the cost of covered services. Out-of-pocket costs are sometimes also called self-pay or direct-pay costs.

Copayments are those patient payments that are required even when there is insurance coverage for eligible service. Deductibles are the patient payment obligations that occur prior to any insurance coverage kicking in. Typical deductibles range from $50 to $200 per person and $100 to $300 per family per year.

When there are no deductibles, an individual is said to have first-dollar coverage. This is extremely rare in the current marketplace.

Deductibles serve two principal functions. One is to eliminate claims obligations for individuals with relatively little annual utilization. The second is to discourage utilization by erecting a financial barrier. Substantial deductibles do have a significant inhibitory effect, although relatively small deductibles have much less impact. Policies sold with very substantial deductibles, perhaps $1,000 to $5,000, provide catastrophic protection.

Premiums drop substantially with such large deductibles, often by as much as 40 percent.

A variation of sorts on high deductible health care coverage is being promoted under the rubric of consumer-driven health care. The idea is that the high deductible provides an incentive for patients to use health care resources more carefully. Such arrangements sometimes also incorporate health savings plans—employers combine a high deductible with pretax withholding of dollars that can be used for various approved health care expenses, again providing an incentive to use resources wisely.

The second category of patient obligation is coinsurance. Coinsurance is a patient payment that occurs concurrently with an insurance company reimbursement or provided service. Coinsurance under indemnity and traditional service insurance is expressed as a percentage of the bill, generally ranging from 10 to 20 percent.

Coinsurance can also be required in a dollar amount rather than as a percentage of the bill. For example, many HMOs, discussed in more detail in the next chapter, require a $5 or $10 copayment at time of service for an office visit. Insurance also serves two functions, the first being to inhibit utilization and the second being to provide revenue. As for deductibles, the larger the coinsurance, the greater its effect in inhibiting utilization.

In indemnity plans, when a patient voluntarily allows the insurance company to pay a claim directly to a provider, such as a hospital, this is termed assignment of benefits. Assignment, however, does not reduce the patient's obligation to pay fees in excess of the allowable indemnity amount, nor does it usually reduce the deductibles or coinsurance.

The premium, or periodic fee for coverage, is computed based on the insurance company's expectation of losses, or claims, plus administrative and operational costs, and profit. As mentioned previously, when the premium is based on the specific experience of the insured group, it is termed to be experience rated. Experience rating results in each group's having its premium based on its historical loss. Experience rating ties the premium to the risk level of the individuals in the group that is being insured. This, combined with higher administrative costs, is a reason why small groups have not been especially attractive to insurance companies.

In community rating, the premium is determined for the entire population, or community, without specific reference to any one subgroup. Thus community rating spreads the risk over a much larger pool, and any one group's experiences do not determine its rate computation. Experience rating has generally been the approach of choice by the insurance industry, but one goal of health care reform is to promote community rating.

An insurance policy remains in force as long as the premium is paid and the contract is valid. Insurance contracts in health care are usually written for six months or one year. The term of the policy may be set for whatever time period the insurance company and the insured agree upon.

Should the premium not be paid, coverage ceases. Most nonhealth policies allow a grace period after the premium is due during which, if the premium is paid up, the policy will remain in force. The grace period usually extends for a short time, often 30 days.

As a contract, an insurance arrangement can be modified. Standard policies are usually modified through the use of a waiver, which contains additional contract terms that differ from the standard contract. In health care, a waiver might stipulate that the policy does not cover a preexisting condition that would otherwise be covered. An insurance company may offer an individual such a policy when the alternative is to refuse to provide any coverage at all.

Most insurance contracts contain numerous terms and conditions. All of these terms are binding. Among the terms and conditions are time limits within which claims must be filed to be considered for payment. Procedures for filing a claim, if applicable, will also be outlined in the contract. Many managed care plans, particularly HMOs, do not require that enrollees file claim forms, a distinct administrative advantage, and another objective of health care reform.

Insurance contracts also usually specify that services are covered only if medically necessary, as determined by the insurer. Services may not be of an experimental nature; they must be part of accepted medical practice.

THE FUTURE OF HEALTH INSURANCE

The health insurance industry is immensely complex, encompassing a huge range of programs, provisions, benefits, and delivery mechanisms. Many organizations provide health care services under a variety of insurance plans and programs. Some are exclusive to one plan or program. Some government agencies such as the Veterans Administration and the United States Military through the Tricare Program also provide forms of insurance programs and plans for designated beneficiaries. Employers provide insurance programs for currently employed individuals as well as in some instances for retirees. The federal government and most state and local governments similarly provide for both active employees and retirees. Health insurance covers a huge range of benefits and services from acute care inpatient and outpatient services to long-term care insurance. The explosion of coverage under managed care plans, discussed in more detail in the next chapter, has further complicated the operating characteristics of the industry. Many federal and state initiatives are directed toward improving insurance coverage and access for individuals or population groups. For example, the federal-state cooperative SCHIP (State Children's Health Insurance Program) initiative has increased Medicaid-related coverage for children of low-income backgrounds without other access to other insurance options. A number of states have developed or are in the process of developing their own insurance initiatives for residents or for population subgroups as well.

Adding to the challenges are a variety of policy initiatives already underway or under consideration for the future. These include, at the extreme, a national health insurance program such as a single-payer effort that would channel all health insurance payment arrangements through a centrally sponsored and organized insurance mechanism. Multiple-payer national plans might also be considered as well. Health savings plans have been experimented with in the past and are currently available for individuals employed in certain settings with specified employer-sponsored health insurance coverage. These plans allow individuals to pay less for their health insurance premiums while saving on a pretax basis funds that can be used for the initial and smaller health care claims, reserving insurance for more serious illness.

Other countries have dealt with health insurance needs in a variety of different ways. The United Kingdom, for example, has a national health care system encompassing nearly all citizens and administered, managed, paid for, and operated essentially by the national government. Canada has a provincial-based health insurance system whereby each province has its own insurance system to pay for the health care needs of its citizens. Many other countries use a combination of patient payment mechanisms and private insurance programs. Unfortunately, the diversity of the international experience does not offer a clear message for the United States, but rather highlights the implications of a variety of options that might be considered.

The rapid growth of managed care, combined with movements toward state, local, and national health care reform, have already greatly changed the face of voluntary insurance. Insurers have dramatically moved to control patients and providers. Open-ended, unmanaged indemnity programs are dinosaurs owing to their lack of control mechanisms.

Most of the large, for-profit insurers involved in health care have repackaged their plans and programs in managed care formats. This allows them greater control over costs and, with national political and policy trends, positions them for the future. Financial pressures on employers prohibit most from offering comprehensive indemnity plans with high premiums, severely stunting any potential for growth in this area. Even entitlement programs have moved toward increasing use of managed care, although evidence of effective cost containment is mixed.

The insurance industry responds to marketplace demand for new products. Over the years this has led to evolving and creative plans for health care services and to new forms of coverage such as for dental and vision care. More recently, there has been a tremendous industry response to the need for long-term care insurance. Long-term care insurance, which may be purchased through employer-sponsored plans or independently through affinity groups, provides protection against the costs of nursing home, home health, and other needs for individuals in the long-term care environment. Long-term care insurance is typically paid for entirely by employees or other enrollees, as the costs are quite substantial. Long-term care products are primarily indemnity oriented, but these plans have become much more sophisticated with many more options in recent years. Exclusion periods, that is how long an individual in need must wait before coverage begins; length of coverage; allowable costs; total benefit packages; and many other variables are now typically considered in the design and selection of long-term care policies. Particularly important are options for inflation protection and for buying coverage far in advance of actual need to allow for a lower premium. In addition, long-term care insurance is highly dependent on adverse risk selection so that individuals cannot obtain coverage once need for care is imminent.

The insurance industry is adept at assessing risks and offering products that reflect current market conditions. The health care industry of the future will require successful insurers to change and adapt. Entitlement programs will also continue to change, reflecting lessons learned elsewhere in the health care industry. The upshot of these trends will be a drastically different, and probably more effective, insurance industry and delivery system, one that will have evolved far from its World War II origins.

STUDY QUESTIONS

1. How are physicians reimbursed?
2. How were hospitals reimbursed by the Medicare program under retrospective reimbursement?
3. How does prospective reimbursement change the incentives for hospitals in the provision of care?
4. What is the nature of the federal Medicare program?
5. How is commercial insurance organized?
6. What is the historical origin of commercial health insurance?
7. In what ways does health insurance not fit the traditional mold of insurance products?
8. What are the differences between group and individual plans?
9. What are the differences between service and indemnity insurance?
10. What is the role of copayments in insurance plans?

CHAPTER 12

Managed Care and the Reorganization of Health Services

Chapter Objectives

1. To describe the historical origins of managed care.
2. To explain the rationale for developing managed care plans and programs.
3. To examine international models of managed care.
4. To explore the historical and philosophical origins of managed care in the United States.
5. To explore the empirical evidence regarding the success of managed care plans in containing health care costs.
6. To define the scope of managed care plans in the United States currently.
7. To discuss the newer and more innovative approaches to organizing managed care services.
8. To depict the mechanisms by which managed care operates.
9. To describe how managed care controls providers and consumers.
10. To identify financial arrangements under managed care, particularly institutional and individual reimbursement mechanisms.
11. To discuss how managed care affects health care delivery organizations.

The dramatic realignment of the relationships between providers, payers, and consumers termed *managed care* encompasses a wide range of incentives and relationships. The fundamental objective of managed care is to restructure the organization of health services in such a manner as to enhance cost containment, maintain quality, and facilitate the management of patient care needs. This chapter traces the history and development of managed care and outlines the methods managed care systems have used in attempts to achieve their objectives.

ORIGINS OF MANAGED CARE

Today's managed care concepts originated with the development, both in the United States and internationally, of prepaid health care plans. Prepayment fundamentally alters the relationships between consumers and providers. The history and current status of managed care plans revolve around substantial changes in how health care systems and services are organized, how providers are paid, and how the relationships between providers, consumers, and insurers (or other payers) are structured. However, from the beginning, managed care has involved much more than just changes in financial incentives. Ultimately, it represents a restructuring of the health care system itself.

A key component of managed care, and of prepayment in general, also includes the administration, monitoring, and feedback mechanisms needed in a "closed" system. Today's managed care arena encompasses a broad array of organizational and managerial approaches to organizing, paying for, and monitoring services.

The Rationale for Managed Care

Fundamentally, managed care operates on the assumption that traditional fee-for-service reimbursement provides inadequate, if any, incentive for cost containment and utilization controls on the part of patients or providers. The need to reorganize financial incentives in such a manner as to discourage excessive utilization, however defined, as well as to provide alternative organizational structures for the provision of care, resulted in the development and evolution of various forms of managed care (Table 12.1).

Managed care represents the broad array of alternative delivery systems and structures that have evolved over the years from the original concepts of prepayment. The term managed care itself is a generic classification for a wide range of organizational and financial arrangements. Managed care, a broad term, is intrinsically not easily defined. From an international perspective, managed care can be found around the globe in various forms, but the methods of delivering care and organizing services vary greatly.

Managed care challenges the commitment of physicians and other providers to the traditional market economy in health care. The challenge is greatest toward fee-for-service, piecework reimbursement, which rewards the quantity of work performed. The early history of prepayment reveals a much different attitude from today's political, social, and economic perspectives.

Historical Development of Managed Care

The origins of managed care can be traced back to a variety of often independent approaches to reor-

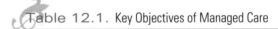

Table 12.1. Key Objectives of Managed Care

Cost containment
Some forms of rationing
Efficiency of care
Less duplication
Administration efficiency
Contracting efficiency
Managing care
Appropriateness of care

ganizing the incentives for providers, and offering a more structured environment for consumers. In the United States, prepaid health care systems represent the earliest forms of managed care.

The Kaiser health care system and Group Health Cooperative of Puget Sound in Seattle, founded by consumers, exemplify early efforts at organizing health care systems that avoided the fee-for-service incentive structure and that focused on organizing patient access to and use of services. These early, prepaid delivery systems, and other closed panel plans, offer a complete system of care to consumers while at the same time radically changing the methods of paying providers. These prepaid systems provide care within a highly structured organization that incorporates financing mechanisms, enrolls a population of consumers, and employs the necessary resources to offer care.

Beginnings in the United States

In the United States, the early prepayment programs focused on *closed panel*, complete delivery systems. These early forms of prepayment were viewed as antithetical to the principles of capitalism that had traditionally been applied to the provision of health care, particularly by private-practice physicians. Physicians employed in prepaid settings were often viewed with suspicion by their colleagues. Local medical societies, as well as the American Medical Association, spoke openly against prepayment and salaried physicians.

This early assault is in stark contrast to the increasing acceptance of the principles of managed care by organized medicine in recent years. Political realities have finally caught up with organized medicine. Changes in the power structure of the health care system have also weakened the power of these special-interest groups.

After World War II, until the early 1970s, relatively limited change occurred in the prepayment arena. Kaiser and a few other large, prepaid delivery systems, mentioned previously, continued their evolutionary growth. A number of other forms of

prepaid health care, most notably medical care foundation plans such as the San Joaquin Foundation, were also developed. Foundation plans were early forms of what subsequently became independent practice associations (IPAs). They were designed to maintain physicians in community-based, fee-for-service practice while using a reimbursement mechanism that allowed for prepayment to the insurer.

HEALTH MAINTENANCE ORGANIZATIONS

The more immediate precursors to today's managed care programs began with the development of health maintenance organizations (HMOs) in the early 1970s. The term *health maintenance organization* was coined by Paul Ellwood, a pediatric neurologist who has long been active in health policy formulation. However, the HMO concept essentially reflected a restatement of many of the established principles of prepayment.

HMOs were formally established through federal legislation during the administration of President Richard M. Nixon. HMOs were an attempt to reorganize health care services to reduce the rate of health care cost increases and to control utilization of services. The Nixon administration viewed HMOs as an adjutant to the wage and price controls that were being utilized at the time to reduce the inflation rate in the general economy.

The federal HMO legislation codified a number of the principles of prepayment and provided incentives for the development of HMOs. Federal, and corresponding state, legislation also required employers to offer employees an HMO option if certain criteria were met. Ironically, many employers today offer only managed care options to their employees. Some HMOs were also given federal financial support for their planning and development.

HMOs were promoted by the administration and the Congress as a private-sector approach to medicine that would control utilization and costs through self-regulation. The legislation reflected a desire to provide comprehensive and good quality services at generally lower total cost than was available in the fee-for-service sector. HMOs were also required to offer a wide range of services, including some preventive care.

Two forms of HMO were originally recognized under the federal legislation, although more exist now. The first was the closed-panel HMO based on a multispecialty group-practice design and typified by Kaiser and Group Health Cooperative of Puget Sound. These plans generally employed their own physicians and paid them a full-time salary, or a salary with incentive compensation, and either owned their own hospitals or contracted for care with local hospitals. Consumers were enrolled in the plan and were offered services solely through the plan's providers.

Closed-panel HMOs have controlled utilization through a number of managed care techniques, such as reliance on primary care gatekeepers. In these organizations, providers generally have less incentive to overutilize specialty services, since compensation is not directly tied to utilization rates. However, the potential for underutilization is a concern.

Independent Practice Associations

The Nixon administration, in an effort to preserve community-based, private medical practice, to allow such practices to share in the proliferation of HMOs, and as a result of political pressures from organized medicine, incorporated a second form of HMO into the federal legislation passed in 1973. This second form, the independent practice plan or association, was modeled on the foundation plans.

Independent practice associations (IPAs) are affiliations of community-based, fee-for-service practitioners who contract to provide care for plan enrollees. The IPA in essence is a risk-taking entity. The IPA contracts with community-based physicians and hospitals for the actual provision of care. The IPA reflects a model of prepayment under which community-based practitioners are geographically disseminated, as opposed to more intensive clustering in larger, multispecialty, closed panel group practices.

IPAs have reimbursed physicians using a number of mechanisms that are also used in some other organizational forms of managed care. These are salary, or a modification of salary using some form of incentive compensation in which the incentive is based on productivity and other factors, such as specialty orientation; capitation, through which the physician is reimbursed a set, monthly fee for all care provided to each enrollee, with the fee determined in some instances by the characteristics of the enrollee, such as age; and finally, fee for service, the least likely mechanism to enhance cost containment. Historically, IPAs have paid physicians primarily through fee-for-service reimbursement, a significant problem when the IPAs themselves are reimbursed based on some form of capitation or monthly premium.

Numerous experiments have been conducted using IPAs and other forms of managed care to reimburse physicians by capitation; capitation is also utilized for reimbursement in the British National Health Service. Under capitation, physicians are provided with an incentive to contain costs, and underutilization may be a problem.

Capitation reimbursement programs have used a variety of mechanisms to offer incentives to physicians. Most notable of these incentives have been pools of reimbursement funds from which capitation payments or, in some instances, fee-for-service payments are withdrawn as utilized, with any funds remaining at the end of the fiscal year being divided between the insurer or employer and the participating physicians as a means of encouraging careful monitoring of utilization. However, these pools have not always provided enough of an incentive to have a substantial effect on utilization patterns.

Historical Economic Performance

Historically, managed care plans have achieved cost containment through reduced hospitalization rates that offset the costs of higher ambulatory care utilization. The increasing use of ambulatory surgery, of outpatient facilities for diagnostic and therapeutic interventions, and of fiberoptic surgical procedures, as well as various forms of rationing, have enhanced the shift from inpatient to outpatient services, particularly in managed care organizations.

Rationing in managed care systems occurs through a number of mechanisms. These include enhanced waiting times to obtain appointments; encouragement of self-care; utilization of the telephone for advising in lieu of in-person visits; reduction in the use of diagnostic procedures and laboratory testing through physician incentives and education; and other constraints on the availability of care for both providers and consumers.

Experience on a macrolevel in constraining the availability of resources, particularly in the British National Health Service, in most of the Canadian provinces, and in the state of Oregon in the United States has been the origin of increased interest in setting budgetary limits for health services at national and system-wide levels. The annual budget process in Kaiser and other closed-panel HMOs also serves the same effect.

It is unlikely that prepaid and managed care programs have actually been able to provide specific units of service at significantly lower per-unit cost than other provider systems. Savings are achieved through reductions in inpatient utilization and through overall constraints on the availability of resources. The relationship between quantity of resources available in a community and utilization of services has long been established. However, quantifying optimal levels of resource availability and relating resources to consumer behavior in a context that promotes quality of care and ensures access have been extremely difficult to achieve.

FURTHER DEVELOPMENT OF MANAGED CARE

The proliferation of managed care programs from the 1980s through 2004 has been dramatic. The Medicare and Medicaid programs are even now embracing managed care. Not only has the number of managed care plans and organizations greatly increased, but the design of prepayment and managed care delivery systems and insurance programs has led to a much greater range of approaches and alternatives.

Closed-panel HMOs continue to be modeled along the original design concepts, although in recent years, governmental mandates regarding the scope of benefits and other constraints have been relaxed. Many HMOs have increased copayments and have expanded their mechanisms for controlling utilization. IPAs have also seen increases in enrollees. IPAs have increasingly focused on contracting with multispecialty group practices as well as on experimentation with alternative approaches to paying physicians to create incentives to contain costs.

The number of HMOs in the nation (Table 12.2) has greatly increased since the 1980s. Many citizens of the United States now receive their health care through some type of structured HMO, although the exact number is difficult to estimate accurately. Many insurance products now represent a form of prepayment or managed care, and the actual number of Americans receiving care under some form of managed care is probably far greater than reflected in the formal count. The Medicare program has also promoted managed care, as has Medicaid. And enrollments are subject to substantial change as employer and consumer preferences change. The federal Balanced Budget Act of 1997 has also promoted experimentation.

Newer Forms of Managed Care

During the 1980s and 1990s, increasing experimentation with various forms of managed care resulted in the development of other models of prepayment. Many of these combine the use of community-based resources with some IPA concepts. Notable among these innovations has been the preferred provider organization (PPO). The PPO is a contracting mechanism that includes fee

Table 12.2. HMOs and Enrollment, Selected Years

Plans and Enrollment	1980	2002
Plans (number)		
All plans	235	500
Model type		
IPA	97	229
Group	138	100
Mixed	—	171
Geographic region		
Northeast	55	87
Midwest	72	140
South	45	178
West	63	95
Enrollment (in thousands)		
Total	9,078	76,100
Model type		
IPA	1,694	31,600
Group	7,384	15,000
Mixed	—	29,600
Federal program		
Medicaid	265	12,800
Medicare	391	5,400

discounting by participating providers and that generally uses community-based practitioners in a modification of the service insurance plans popular in the 1960s and 1970s.

In a PPO, the sponsor, such as an insurance company, establishes contracts with participating networks of providers, including hospitals and physicians. The physicians may be in multispecialty or single-specialty groups. The providers offer services to enrollees in the PPO in exchange for reimbursement based on a discounted, contracted, prenegotiated fee basis, using a fee schedule for specific procedures, or on a bundled-services basis. Reimbursement is often based on previously established, usual and customary fees, with a discount applied by the PPO. PPO contracts may include requirements for utilization review.

Enrollees in the PPO must use contracted providers to obtain maximum benefits under the plan. Services obtained from nonparticipating providers are reimbursed at substantially lower levels in an indemnity format. Noncovered services are not reimbursed at all. For services that are covered and for which care was obtained from a nonparticipating provider, the consumer is also at risk for fees in excess of the usual and customary fee schedule.

PPOs usually require a deductible on a per-person and per-family basis, as well as a copayment of 10 to 20 percent of allowable charges for covered services provided by participating physicians and other providers. Inpatient and certain other services may be covered at 100 percent. Some services, such as pharmacy, may require a separate copayment as well. PPOs typically require a 30- or 40-percent copayment for services provided by nonparticipating providers.

The *point-of-service* (POS) plan allows some out-of-plan use within the HMO format. Enrollees can elect a nonplan provider at the point of service and with much higher copayments.

Many new forms of managed care and HMOs, including direct contract, have been developed. The operational principles of many models have also changed over time to adapt to a changing health care environment.

Managed care truly represents an evolving concept, one that is likely to adapt to changes in economic and political realities. In recent years, a primarily consumer-led backlash against certain managed care provisions perceived as unduly limiting patient freedom and provider access has led to some loosening up in the provisions of managed care arrangements. Managed care essentially represents a more modern and economically rational response to traditional indemnity insurance approaches, recognizing the unrealistic and relatively open-ended nature of indemnity in light of increasing health care costs. Managed care will continue to evolve with the addition and deletion of various incentives and disincentives for consumers and providers. Managed care is a dynamic process both in its evolution and in its daily operation. As a result, it is essential to understand the underlying principles of managed care and how various mechanisms can be utilized to implement these plans.

PRINCIPLES OF MANAGED CARE

Managed care focuses on the relationships among payers, providers, and consumers. Many important and not fully validated concepts have been developed to influence, monitor, and control these relationships. Since managed care evolved from prepayment and from a recognition that open-ended, relatively unstructured, approaches to health care delivery lead to excessive utilization, duplication, wasted services, and possibly lower quality, managed care is built on the premise that more formal structuring of the system is essential.

Incentives for providers and consumers must enhance their efficient use of services. These mechanisms impact quality, access, and cost of services. These mechanisms also threaten many traditional values, such as free choice of providers by consumers, unlimited access to care, direct consumer access for specialty services, and provider freedom in responding to patient needs.

Primary Care Gatekeepers

One of the most important, and controversial, control mechanisms used in managed care is the primary care physician *gatekeeper*. The gatekeeper should be an informed patient advocate serving two roles in the provision of health services. First, the gatekeeper serves as the physician for the ongoing primary care needs of the consumer. In this role, this physician, who is typically a family practitioner, general internist, pediatrician, or, in some instances, obstetrician/gynecologist, provides as many primary care services as he or she is capable of consistent with the provider's clinical skills. The gatekeeper is intended to be the most cost-efficient provider of primary care services and the one who is most responsive to a patient's immediate needs.

The second key role of the gatekeeper is to be a manager of the patient's medical care needs. The gatekeeper is clinically knowledgeable and familiar with the patient's needs. The gatekeeper can direct the patient to other specialized resources. Referral to specialists occurs only with the approval of the gatekeeper.

The gatekeeper in managed care can successfully reduce some costs. However, gatekeepers also incur a variety of costs, such as extra visits to assess needs, follow-up requirements after specialty referral, delays in care resulting from the gatekeeper process, impacts on patient and provider satisfaction, and administrative costs.

Ideally, the gatekeeper serves as a patient advisor and provides oversight and a coordinating role. The gatekeeper should reduce duplication of services. Depending on how the gatekeeper is reimbursed, there may be incentives for under- or overutilization of specialists, and thus the gatekeeper may add rationing as well as rationalization to the system.

Other Controls Over Utilization of Services

In addition to the gatekeeper, managed care relies on various other forms of utilization review and quality assurance. The mechanisms used vary from plan to plan, but they revolve around similar concepts.

The principal objective of utilization review in managed care plans is to monitor and control the use of services and to determine the appropriateness of the care that is provided. Utilization review is also used to inhibit utilization through such mechanisms as prior authorization.

Prior authorization is utilized in managed care for such elective surgical procedures as appendectomy and hysterectomy. Prior authorization usually consists of review by consulting nurses and/or physicians (employed by the payer), who assess clinical criteria for the proposed procedure and judge appropriateness.

Second-opinion surgical programs also may be required. Under these programs a second clinician in the same surgical specialty will review the patient and independently determine the appropriateness of the proposed procedure.

Provider Networks

Managed care relies on institutional and individual providers who have a contractual arrangement with the payer. The contractual arrangements structure the delivery system. These arrangements are based on contractual requirements for defining where and how care is provided and for monitoring such care. The structure of these relationships can vary tremendously depending on the type of managed care. Closed-panel, multispecialty group practice-based plans, such as Kaiser, rely on direct employment of providers.

Managed care organizations contract with local providers establishing networks of providers. Network participants provide services to eligible enrollees in the plan. Providers are reimbursed based on contractual mechanisms such as capitation, some modification of fee for service, negotiated and discounted fee schedules, or bundled packages.

Managed care plans have increasingly contracted with large, multispecialty medical groups that offer a wide range of services and reduced administrative complexity. Physicians, and other providers, may be dropped from networks because of high costs and questions regarding quality of care and patient satisfaction.

The plan includes a provider services department that signs up, retains, and monitors participating practitioners. Management information systems process claims and utilization data, and possibly patient satisfaction surveys, physician and hospital registries, referral sources for specialty services, and other key elements of information.

Consumers are provided with limited information (e.g., address, specialty) on network providers. Participating physicians may cap practice enrollments to avoid excess patient demand. The eligible enrollees cared for by an individual provider, particularly in primary care, are termed a panel of patients (physicians in a closed-panel HMO are a panel of providers). The characteristics of the panel largely define need for services based on age distribution, disease, and illness levels. In plans that rely on capitation, equitable distribution of patients among providers by intensity of need, or adjustment of capitation reimbursement to reflect intensity, may be required.

Networks generally differentiate between primary care providers and specialty services. Specialists are under contract based on referral from primary care physicians and may be paid by capitation or fee for service.

MANAGEMENT OF THE CONSUMER

Managed care networks emphasize managing consumer use of the health care system through incentives, disincentives, and monitoring. Consumer controls on use of services include financial and operational mechanisms.

Financial Incentives

Financial mechanisms include copayments and deductibles. HMOs use these mechanisms the least, and PPO-type plans use them the most. Financial controls targeted at providers include discounts on fees and bundling of multiple services into individual packages.

Financial controls on consumers tend to be weaker in managed care plans than those on providers, although the onus on the consumer will likely increase in the future. Financial barriers ideally reduce medically unnecessary elective visits and procedures but avoid discouraging urgent and emergency care.

Nonfinancial Incentives

Nonfinancial incentives and disincentives in managed care plans are important in affecting use of services and in channeling patients into established networks. Nonfinancial incentives include structuring the network to require the use of participating providers for full coverage, authorization for hospital admission and for selected elective surgical procedures, and controlled referral to specialists and ancillary services.

The payer may operate these control mechanisms him/herself or, particularly in employer-sponsored plans, may contract with a third-party administrator (TPA) or utilization management firm. Increasingly sophisticated computer programs, combined with highly trained staff and clinical algorithms, are often capable of making reasonable judgments about the appropriateness of care.

Managed care programs, particularly closed-panel HMOs, also utilize structural impediments to ration resources, as mentioned earlier. These include waiting times for appointments, reliance on telephone and e-mail consultation, and patient education for self-care.

Case Management

Case management and other aggressive interventions channel patient use of services for more serious illnesses. Case management, in which the patient's health care needs, progress, and use of services are monitored and controlled by a specially trained individual, often a nurse, targets the use of expensive (and especially tertiary) care. Quality of care can be improved through better coordination of services, reduced duplication, and more effective and rapid access to specialty care. Case management may encourage the use of home health care and other alternatives to institutional care.

Patients with complex acute, or serious chronic, disease are suitable for case management. Case managers, as experienced and knowledgeable professionals, can alleviate patient fears regarding appropriateness of care and facilitate access to needed services.

Administration of Managed Care Programs

Managed care programs can reduce administrative overhead. HMOs, particularly the closed-panel form, may eliminate the need for claims forms and other administrative burdens. Reimbursement of providers based on capitation or salary also reduces the administrative burden for filing claims. Fee-for-service-oriented PPOs and IPAs, however, may still require extensive paperwork because of the need to file claims. Reduction in paperwork and administrative costs using managed care is an admirable objective for health care reform.

Managed care does incur administrative costs because of required monitoring of care, utilization review, and consumer relations. Recording transactions is valuable to determine utilization patterns and to assess appropriateness of care. In the absence of these administrative systems, patient and provider assessments of utilization and quality are much more difficult to obtain.

The National Committee for Quality Assurance (NCQA), a nonprofit organization based in Washington, DC, provides a platform for the voluntary accreditation of health plans. Participating plans are evaluated across a range of criteria and the results of the assessments are available to consumers through the organization's Web site and publications. Participation in this voluntary accreditation requires data collection and reporting but also establishes a plan's compliance with a set of specific evaluation criteria. Overall, in a significant movement toward various forms of assessment and evaluation of health plans and their member organizations is gaining steam, with support and encouragement and in some cases, mandates from various levels of government and a variety of nonprofit organizations. These efforts empower employers, consumers, and government to establish and eventually raise the bar on minimum levels of quality expected from provider organizations and insurance plans.

Most managed care programs require a membership department to deal with consumer administrative problems as well as to address patient complaints. Many managed care programs utilize compulsory arbitration for risk management.

Benefit packages may be broader under managed care, especially for preventive services such as routine physical examinations, vision and hearing screening, well-child care, and patient education. The ability of managed care networks to contract with providers at significantly discounted rates may also allow for a broader scope of services.

Managed care programs have struggled with balancing greater access to a broader array of benefits while at the same time gaining a competitive advantage from their reduced total costs of services. Defining a minimum benefit package under federal entitlement programs is particularly germane to assessing the scope of benefits that can be provided in a cost-effective manner under managed care programs. A commitment to preventive services, particularly those that have been analytically demonstrated to provide population-based benefits, will be an important component of national health policy. Providing incentives for plans to take a long-term perspective will also eventually lead to lower health care costs.

FINANCIAL ARRANGEMENTS UNDER MANAGED CARE

Managed care structures the provision of services in a more controlled and organized manner than the traditional fee-for-service mechanisms of financing and reimbursement. Consumer incentives are designed to create financial barriers to access, although these are typically minimal in these plans. For many provider organizations, reimbursement mechanisms under most forms of managed care represent a radical change from traditional, fee-for-service-dominated methods.

Provider Reimbursement Issues

In most fee-for-service indemnity insurance plans, as discussed in Chapter 11, physicians and hospitals are paid by the patient; then, the patient is reimbursed by his or her insurer or employer based on the terms of the insurance plan. Some form of fee schedule is used. In the most traditional fee-for-service plans, reimbursement of physicians and other individuals is based on usual, customary, and reasonable (UCR) negotiated, and sometimes discounted, fees. Institutional providers are usually reimbursed based on negotiated per-diem or per-admission diagnosis-related fees.

Some managed care programs, such as PPOs and some IPAs, follow the fee-for-service-based UCR service reimbursement approach. However, provider discounts of UCR fees may be greater than under a traditional service plan. The failure to bundle services, or to use capitation or other arrangements with incentives for reduced utilization, is a severe hindrance to containing costs in these forms of managed care.

A key objective of managed care is to shift the financial risk onto the provider as an incentive toward cost containment and appropriate resource utilization. Financial risk pools serve to share risk. Under these pools, reimbursement for a group of patients is put into one or two pots, combining or separately funding inpatient and outpatient services. Dollars are drawn from each pool to meet patient needs, including referral to specialists and inpatient services. Funds remaining in the pool at the end of a defined time period are then divided between payers and providers. The potential for additional profit creates an incentive to control expenditures.

Risk-sharing pools can present some problems, including determining how large a pool must be to have significant psychological and economic impact; the potential for underutilization and hence lower quality of care; the way pools should be structured and what services are appropriately included or excluded; and the extent to which funds remaining in the pools should be shared between providers and payers. All risk-sharing arrangements involve serious concern about their effects on physician judgment and the difficulty of ensuring appropriate medical care.

Another complex issue is medical malpractice. Some utilization is attributable to the practice of "defensive" medicine. This is the attempt to ensure that the practitioner provides all care that other community physicians would have provided in their best clinical and professional judgment. Patients must be able to redress their grievances. How this can be most fairly dealt with under managed care needs further attention.

Finally, patients expect medical personnel to find and solve their problems. Patient expectations rarely consider cost containment or rationing. Patients frequently complain that physicians do not spend adequate time with them, that they are rushed through visits, or that conditions and treatments are not adequately explained. Patient expectations must be balanced against economic efficiency.

MANAGED CARE AND DELIVERY ORGANIZATIONS

Managed care has profound effects on health care delivery organizations. Managed care contracts impose complex requirements on providers, such as those for information systems, accounting for care, and quality assurance.

Management information system needs can be complex under managed care plans. Managed care contracts typically specify reporting requirements, such as utilization of services and quality assurance. Information requirements vary considerably depending on the sponsoring insurer or employer and on the type of plan. In contrast, traditional indemnity plans require little, if any, reporting.

Managed care contracts may require review of provider qualifications, such as physician specialty board eligibility or certification, licensure, and disciplinary actions. Contracts can specify quality assurance activities that must be conducted and for which reports must be provided. Contract requirements may specify the maintenance and reporting of enrollee characteristics, health services utilization, patient complaints, and other indicators of the use of services. Financial information may be required to verify the fiscal viability of the provider organization. Institutional licensure and other characteristics may be a requirement of the contract and must be reported on a periodic basis.

Provider Arrangements and Affiliations

The evolution of managed care in the United States has led to much more extensive interprovider and interinstitutional arrangements than have traditionally existed in the health care system. Hospitals and physicians, hospitals and other provider organizations, hospitals and hospitals, and physicians and physicians have increasingly formed alliances of various sorts to provide a basis for contracting with payers. These alliances have taken many legal and organizational forms.

Hospitals have purchased group practices and other components of the health care system to form an integrated delivery system for purposes of contracting. Hospital systems, and alliances of hospitals and hospital systems, have evolved to achieve economies of scale as well as for contracting purposes. Independent practice association-types of affiliations have been formed to provide a basis for individual physicians to contract with payers.

The increasing dependence of the health care system on these alliances has led to a significant trend away from the role of the physician practice as an independent, entrepreneurial unit. Physicians and other providers have become increasingly dependent on each other, leading to numerous sources of stress and interorganizational conflict. Questions as to who determines the basis for contracting and who negotiates the specific terms of the contracts are frequently raised in these affiliation arrangements. The role and power of the hospital versus its medical staff is a particularly important issue. In general, in managed care arrangements, physicians have lost power and prestige.

In some cities, such as Rochester, New York; Minneapolis, Minnesota; and San Diego, California, economic pressures have led to substantial consolidation of providers and to the development of competing health care systems. Some of these systems have developed their own managed care products. Vertically integrated health care systems raise issues of competition and antitrust, fiscal viability, the role of for-profit versus not-for-profit organizations, the independent identity of medical staffs, and many other exceedingly complex concerns, many of which are discussed elsewhere in this book.

The complexities of physician incentive arrangements include the need to promote productivity and efficiency in the provision of care. Differences between productivity of surgeons in prepaid organizations versus those in fee-for-service practice, for example, suggest the potential for much greater productivity under managed care. Higher productivity leads to reduced per-unit fees while maintaining provider income but requires that providers work longer and more intensive hours. This raises other issues about provider income expectations, willingness to work harder for the same or slightly enhanced pay, and quality of care under conditions of higher workloads.

Provider economic incentives and pressures may result in physician interactions with patients that may be less satisfactory for both parties and more bureaucratic. Physicians may feel that under managed care payers are micromanaging the clinical process. Physician autonomy has declined under managed care; this decline is at least lamented, if not resented, by most physicians. The implications for the nation's health care system of low physician morale, increased work loads, and monitoring and control of clinical services must be carefully considered.

Risk sharing may threaten the solvency of some institutions and organizations. With provider organizations assuming more risk, there is a potential for premium rate miscalculation and for adverse-risk selection that could lead to serious fiscal losses.

Stop-loss insurance coverage and assumption of risk through other reinsurance mechanisms can help alleviate these concerns.

The insolvency of some of the early IPAs focused attention on difficulties inherent in reimbursing physicians. More recently, some large insurers have faced financial problems from their involvement in the health care industry owing to inadequate controls on utilization and errant actuarial assumptions.

Managed care contracts offer leverage for both significant profits and substantial losses. Managed care contracts must allow for reasonable profits, avoid underutilization and price gouging, and strike many other balances.

Finally, from a financial perspective, comprehensive risk management is essential. Risk management must include control of medical malpractice risk, including the utilization of compulsory arbitration to reduce litigation costs, patient satisfaction surveys and other efforts to assess consumer satisfaction, general liability protection, and fiscal and utilization monitoring and controls to assure fiscal stability. The financial well-being of the nation's health care system is dependent on the fiscal viability of providers and payers. Reimbursement mechanisms must acknowledge the need for solvency within the system.

CONSUMER PERSPECTIVES ON MANAGED CARE

Managed care systems present an array of challenges for the consumer. In selecting from alternative managed care systems, the consumer must weigh numerous factors. These include potential constraints on utilization associated with waiting times, limited access to specialty services, and other effects from an overburdened system, or one intentionally rationing services.

Depending on the provider's incentives, physicians may not appear responsive to patients. Satisfying patient desires may be a lower priority in managed care than in fee-for-service and indemnity plans.

Advantages for the Consumer

Managed care has many attributes for consumers. Coverage of services is broader, and the financial obligation on the part of the patient is usually lower in managed care plans. Managed care plans also usually require less consumer paperwork. Consumers face a more defined system that reduces the need for second-guessing and for confusing choices.

On balance, managed care plans are advantageous for consumers seeking an organized delivery system, desiring broader benefits and lower out-of-pocket costs, and who are relatively indifferent to externally imposed constraints. Managed care tends to be less desirable for patients who are not price sensitive, who want a broader array of choices, and who seek more involvement in directing their own care.

STUDY QUESTIONS

1. What are the historical bases for today's managed care plans?

2. What is the rationale for the development of managed care in the United States?

3. What international examples highlight the use of managed care principles in other countries?

4. How did health maintenance organizations get their start?

5. What has been the success of managed care plans thus far in the United States?

6. What are preferred provider organizations, exclusive provider organizations, and point-of-service plans?

7. What is the role of the primary care gatekeeper in managed care programs?

8. How do managed care plans put together their provider networks?

9. How do managed care plans control the use of health care services by consumers?

10. How do managed care programs control physician practice patterns?

11. What are the advantages and disadvantages of managed care from a policy perspective?

12. What is the impact of managed care on health care delivery organizations?

CHAPTER 13

Regulating and Planning for the System

Chapter Objectives

1. To describe the history of health care planning in the United States.
2. To describe the history of health care regulation in the United States.
3. To explain the rationale underlying regionalization, particularly in comparison to competitive markets.
4. To discuss the rationale for governmental intervention in the health care system and the specific mechanisms used by government.

Over the years, planning and regulatory mechanisms imposed by government, payers, and others have affected the way the health care system operates. This chapter describes and analyzes the history of these efforts. An understanding of our past efforts will help us analyze current and future proposals for intervention in the system.

The mixed success, and frequent failure, of these efforts has brought us to today's initiatives for health care reform. Of course, we tried to reform our nation's health care system for most of the twentieth century. The wording in the Report of the Committee on the Cost of Medical Care published in the early 1900s under the auspices of, among others, the American Medical Association, sounds suspiciously like our current debate.

We have tried many piecemeal approaches to changing the system—and, to this day, we do not have concurrence on what works best.

PLANNING HEALTH CARE SERVICES

Political and economic forces have shaped our approaches to planning and regulating the health care system. Over the years, we have gravitated from one approach to another, largely as a result of the national political environment at the time.

Our nation is at odds with much of the developed world in that we still have not adequately addressed issues of universal access to care and the right to minimum benefits. The vital nature of health care suggests that our nation should have solved these problems long ago, but the political forces that shape national health policy inhibited resolution of these issues.

Regionalization

From an international perspective, many countries have moved toward national health systems in some form. Examples include the United Kingdom's National Health Service and Sweden's highly organized system.

In the United States, examples of integrated systems include the Kaiser and other closed-panel group-practice health maintenance organizations (HMOs). The military health care system is another example.

Centrally controlled health care systems, including some managed care plans, utilize regionalization for health planning and resource allocation. Characteristics of regionalization are listed in Table 13.1. Under regionalization, resources are allocated geographically and to population groups based on actual need as determined by careful health planning. Populations are enrolled in the

Table 13.1. Concepts of Regionalization

Area	Regionalization Requirement
Service population	Defined geographically or by enrollment Health care needs identifiable for planning Target population
System characteristics	Coordinated, systematic networks Integrated care Primary care-based with specialty referrals Decentralized decision making Shared services Regional planning based on need
Planning and resource allocation	Dynamic system Prospective budgeting based on need Utilization controls Assured access Adequate information for planning Cooperation, not competition
Organization structure	Decentralized decision making Systemwide superstructure Consumer accountability

plan and usually assigned to a primary care physician, often using the gatekeeper mechanism.

Under regionalization, local community hospital beds are also allocated based on population size and health care needs. Local hospitals feed into regional and tertiary care hospitals. Only the facilities absolutely needed for a community are built.

Physicians are allocated panels of patients with referrals, as needed, for specialty care. Often, specialists are assigned to work at the hospitals. Rather than a system where each hospital tries to have a complete range of services, resources are strictly allocated so that a community has only what it needs for its population. This reduces duplication. Control of the system means controlling resource allocation, using budgeting, and managing the patient.

Regionalizing all services in the United States might be achieved by consolidating all health care facilities and forming a single, unified system with central control. Duplicative resources would be moved to ensure geographic coverage. Considerable consolidation of health care resources and systems is currently under way in the industry, especially in the private sector. This market force is leading to more rationalization in some communities. Increasing competition and pricing pressures will encourage this trend in the future.

HEALTH PLANNING IN AMERICA

Our nation has tried health planning to promote more efficiency in the system, although these efforts have met with only very limited success. In the United States, voluntary health planning traces its origins back to the 1940s when hospital councils were established in various cities, notably New York.

Hospital councils, many of which exist today, promoted limited voluntary health planning among their members. Hospitals agreed to share or consolidate services or might trade off the closure of one service, such as pediatrics, in one hospital in exchange for expansion of another service, such as emergency care. Shared services included such items as laundry and management information systems in the days of the large mainframe.

By and large, these early voluntary health planning efforts made little contribution to economic efficiency and improved patient access to services. Voluntary health planning is limited by each institution's own goals, self-protection, and unwillingness to give up much for the benefit of the larger community.

Health planning was given a further boost in the late 1940s with the passage of the Hill–Burton legislation. Hill–Burton promoted hospital development and renovation after World War II. During the war, the nation's resources were allocated to the war effort, and, as a result, many hospital facilities became depleted and needed renovation. In addition, after the war, there was a great expansion of the suburbs of many cities; these areas needed all kinds of infrastructure, including hospitals.

The Hill–Burton legislation mandated that the states compute bed-to-population ratios to determine where new hospital beds were needed. This federal mandate was required prior to the allocation of funds for hospital construction and renovation. Although the approach to health planning that this law required was simplistic, Hill–Burton did mark a significant federal initiative to rationalize allocation of resources in the health care industry.

With the passage of Medicare and Medicaid during the 1960s, and the great emphasis on social services and access to care under the Great Society of President Lyndon B. Johnson, the federal government became increasingly involved in health care planning. Recognizing the increasing dollars that the federal government was putting into health care through entitlement programs, Congress believed that it had the right to demand that the system be operated more efficiently. Political realities, however, limited federal intervention.

The federal government mandated regional health planning through the establishment of local and statewide health planning agencies under the Community and Health Resources Development

Act of 1965. This act created agencies throughout the country called the Community Health Planning (known as b) agencies and statewide, Community Health Planning (known as a), coordinating agencies. These agencies assessed local health care needs and advocated enhanced efficiency, coordination, and distribution of resources. However, these agencies had little or no actual regulatory power and were largely ineffective.

The CHP agencies were eliminated with the passage of the Health Planning and Resources Development Act of 1974, an attempt to reformulate the nation's approach to voluntary health planning. This act created new, local health systems agencies and, again, state-wide agencies to oversee the activities of the voluntary, local agencies in each state. As for the earlier legislation, various community and national advisory panels provided an avenue for consumer and professional involvement. The health systems agencies prepared an inventory of each community's health care resources. An annual implementation plan detailed needed changes in health care resources for each community.

Recognizing that voluntary planning is unlikely to result in rationalization of the system, many states enacted Certificate of Need legislation, which still exists in some states today. Certificate of Need required regulatory approval before expansion or construction of major health care facilities and services. The size of expansion projects requiring approval varied from state to state and also changed over time.

Certificate of Need applied only to new services or construction, essentially grandfathering in all existing resources. In addition, Certificate of Need was influenced by politics so that some providers, usually hospitals, were able to use appeals and political persuasion with state legislatures to circumvent these restrictions. Certificate of Need has also been administratively cumbersome.

The evidence suggests that Certificate of Need has had minimal impact on resource allocation. Many providers redirected capital dollars to unreg-

ulated areas to avoid this regulation. With its limited scope and its inability to substantially alter the array of preexisting resources, Certificate of Need did not even apply to most services.

Concurrent with Certificate of Need, the federal government enacted Section 1122 of the Social Security Act Amendments, which required Medicare fund recipients to comply with state Certificate of Need laws. A health care facility that did not comply with Certificate of Need had its Medicare reimbursement reduced by an amount proportional to the amount of the illegal construction or service.

To give the health planning agencies some teeth, Certificate of Need reviews were conducted under the authority of the local health systems agencies. These reviews were advisory to the state agencies, which had ultimate decision-making authority. The health planning agencies used their assessments of local health care resources to determine the appropriateness of new projects. Between the voluntary efforts of the local agencies and the mandated reviews under Certificate of Need, many agencies were able to have some influence over the development of new resources, but the impact of these efforts was negligible nationally.

OTHER FORMS OF INTERVENTION

Other planning and regulatory efforts in the health care industry are summarized in Table 13.2. These regulatory interventions have targeted both individuals and institutions.

Regulatory intervention aimed at individuals include licensure of professionals, such as physicians and nurses, grants to individuals to pursue health professions training, and income tax benefits for health care utilization. The federal government has allowed the deductibility of certain health care expenses on federal income tax returns, which has the effect of subsidizing the industry. Since 1986, the scope of deductible items has been reduced to

Table 13.2. Selected Regulatory Mechanisms

Regulation Category	Individuals	Institutions

Subsidies	Supply
	  Training grants
	
	Demand
	  Medicare/Medicaid
	  Tax exemptions/credits
	  Entitlement programs
		Supply
		  Construction grants, loans, loan guarantees
		Tax exemptions
		
		Demand
		  Tax exemptions to employers

Entry restrictions	Personnel licensure	Facilities licensure Capital expenditure controls
Rate controls	Fee schedules	Rate-setting commissions Medicare prospective payment reimbursement
Quality controls	Professional review organizations Utilization review Preadmission authorization Second-opinion surgery reviews	Certification for Medicare and Medicaid

the point where few individual taxpayers are now able to avail themselves of these subsidies.

Another tax advantage has been the nontaxability of health insurance benefits provided by employers. Since premiums paid by an employer can be substantial, this benefit has great monetary value to employees.

Market interventions by government regulators aimed at individuals also include medical specialty board certification and certification of other professionals. Licensure is a governmental function, but certification is generally performed by private, not-for-profit entities, such as medical specialty boards.

Regulatory interventions aimed at institutions include, at the local level, health and safety codes, which are quite strict for hospitals and nursing homes. Building codes, zoning regulations, and other local rules also affect the health care industry.

Institutional regulatory intervention also involves the tax code. For employers, health care benefits purchased on behalf of employees are a tax-deductible, hence subsidized, expense. Health care organizations that operate as nonprofit enti-

ties do not pay taxes, another form of subsidization. Subsidies for facilities construction have included Hill–Burton, municipal bond borrowing authority, and grants for education and research.

Insurance and reimbursement arrangements, by their nature, are themselves regulatory mechanisms. Entitlement programs, Medicare in particular, have used a heavy hand in influencing the health care system, using reimbursement policy. The conditions under which reimbursement is paid for and authorized such as bundling of services, fees, and emphasizing outpatient services dramatically affect health care.

An excellent example of the impact of reimbursement policy as a form of regulation is the prospect of payment system implemented by Medicare for hospital reimbursement. Under this plan, currently in effect, hospitals are paid prospectively rather than after the fact, based essentially on a preestablished schedule of fees so that hospitals have an incentive to be more efficient in the delivery of services. Payment mechanisms have been and will continue to be an extremely effective avenue for impacting individual and organizational patterns within the nation's health care system. The more recent move toward consumer-directed health plans presumably will provide some of these powers to patients as they increasingly assume more responsibility in directing their own patterns of care. However, historically, patients have been much less able to influence or control the operation of health care organizations than have been payers and government.

Direct controls over hospital budgets and fees have also been mandated. Hospital rate-setting commissions have operated in the states of Washington and Maryland, among others. Commissions set hospital budgets or fees prospectively. Rate-setting commissions were implemented to moderate health care cost inflation, but their overall success has been rather limited. In addition, the costs of regulation have to be weighed against traditional market results as an alternative.

Under the Medicare program, the federal government stipulates that hospitals, nursing homes, and certain other providers be certified to receive reimbursement. Certification is based on an assessment of the institution's compliance with various regulations.

The voluntary accreditation of hospitals, ambulatory care, and other providers is sponsored by the Joint Commission on the Accreditation of Health Care Organizations and other voluntary, not-for-profit accrediting agencies. Most hospitals are accredited by the Joint Commission, and many ambulatory surgery centers and group practices are accredited by one of the specialized accrediting organizations. Accreditation and certification help ensure a minimum level of quality, but they can also serve as a barrier to entry for new competitors.

THE FUTURE OF CONTROLS

Our attempts to regulate, manage, and control the health care system have had mixed success. Many regulations have some significant impact, but at a cost. The increase in administrative complexity and the decrease in physician autonomy are valid concerns for the future. Managed care uses many of these mechanisms, as well. Finally, reimbursement policies also greatly affect the way the system is operated and controlled.

Our efforts to control, regulate, and manage the health care system through voluntary and governmental initiatives have brought us to the doorstep of health care reform. The continuing evolution of our technology for assessing and controlling the system has improved our ability to achieve specific goals related to access, quality, and utilization of services. However, strategic and organizational planning conducted within each organization has been very effective in competitive markets from an institutional, but not necessarily community, perspective. These efforts have expanded in recent years with an emphasis on organizational goals and missions, marketing, and competitive strategy.

Control over certain aspects of the nation's health care system is improving and will continue to improve in the future. Quality and utilization of services, also discussed in detail in the next chapter of this book, is receiving considerable attention with the likelihood that current responses will substantially improve the quality and utilization controls. The increasing use of computerized medical records within the health care system, which is finally gaining considerable momentum after many false starts, is likely to offer a platform for much better monitoring and control of health care services. Political and economic pressures within the system and from payers to further improve quality is also now having a much more significant impact on delivery of care and the behavior of providers. Pressures to gain operational efficiencies, a trend over the past decade in the rest of the nation's economy, particularly under pressure from increased competition and an international marketplace, is finally making its way more substantially into the health care arena as well. Vast opportunities exist and will be taken advantage of to improve the operational efficiency of the health care system as well as to better coordinate and improve the quality of the clinical care provided.

As a nation, we have failed to "pull it all together" into a cohesive, unified approach to the delivery of health care services for all Americans. Where we stand and the directions and challenges that face us for the future, including quality of care and national health policy issues, are subjects that will be discussed in the remaining chapters of this book.

STUDY QUESTIONS

1. What were the origins of health planning in the United States?
2. In what ways does regionalization force a national allocation of resources in a health care system?
3. What regulatory mechanisms are targeted toward individuals?
4. What regulatory mechanisms are targeted toward institutions?

CHAPTER 14

Quality of Care

Chapter Objectives

1. To discuss mechanisms for measuring quality assessment and assurance services.
2. To examine what quality means.
3. To interpret the system's role in assuring quality.

We all seek the highest quality health care we can find, but how do we measure quality? This is an extremely complicated question. There are many answers to this question, but none is ideal.

In recent years, considerable attention has been directed toward medical errors and other examples of inefficiency, poor practice, hypergenic disease, inefficiencies, and incompetancies within the nation's health care system. While the previous chapter addressed avenues of intervention directed at the overall operation of the system itself, this chapter focuses more on the specific delivery of medical and surgical and avenues for measuring that interaction and improving the overall nature of that transaction. In addition, for many years, considerable evidence has evolved questioning lack of uniformity of health care services across the country with vastly different rates of surgical procedures, different utilization of resources, and differences in approaches to clinical situations clearly in evidence from a variety of studies comparing different geographic regions. These peculiar results further raised issues about the appropriateness of health care clinical services throughout the country. Malpractice concerns, clinical competency, and even patient responsibility for compliance with medical regimens add to a long list of quality-related issues to be addressed by the nation's health care system for today and for the future. Add in also, a variety of mandates from various levels of government, such as those in certain states that mandate nurse to patient staffing ratios and the complexity of measuring and assuring the quality of care becomes increasingly difficult to attain.

QUALITY ASSESSMENT AND ASSURANCE

Quality of care is a measure or indicator of the level of performance of the provider in comparison to some set of expectations or standards. The reality is that measuring quality is an extremely difficult task. Relating quality measures to what happens to patients, especially on an ongoing basis, is one of our greatest challenges in measuring, monitoring, and managing health care services.

Quality Assessment

Quality assessment is the process of measuring the quality of care provided in a health care setting. Traditionally, quality of health care is measured using three criteria areas: structure, process, and outcome.

The structural assessment of quality focuses on the environment within which services are provided. Structure includes such factors as compliance with health and safety codes, having appropriate committee meetings of the medical staff so that there is adequate oversight, having the right equipment, and employing staff who are correctly educated and certified, and whose performance is routinely monitored. Accreditation historically emphasized structural aspects of quality, since they are among the easier measures to evaluate, but is now moving into outcomes measurement.

The process of care measures what is done to the patient and its appropriateness. Process measures include tests and procedures performed, evaluations of patients, therapies instituted, and other elements of the care process. Process of care is also relatively easy to measure, generally relying on the medical record as the principal source of data.

Relating process to how well the patient responds is more complex. Process is usually evaluated against protocols distributed by professional associations and medical societies. The degree of compliance with these protocols determines how appropriate the process of care is.

For example, a child coming into a doctor's office with an earache might be expected, based on established protocols, to have specific tests performed and, if the tests so indicate, to have a type of medicine prescribed. Quality assessment teams might pull the records of all patients with that presenting problem and determine the degree to which each physician's patients had the appropriate tests performed and the correct medication prescribed.

Outcome measures of the quality of care are perhaps the most important but, at the same time, the most difficult to perform. Outcome measures examine the results of the care process. Among the outcome measures typically used are morbidity, including infection rates, mortality, and functional status.

Relating outcomes to the structure and process of care is difficult. Outcomes are the result of the care process as well as of the physiological and psychological composition of the patient. Patient compliance with medical regimens, which is notoriously bad in many populations, might mean, for example, that the medical regimen would have led to the right outcome if the patient had done what he or she was told to do. Oftentimes, the provider is not even aware of patient's failure to follow medical orders.

Many factors beyond the provider's control, such as physiological and biological considerations, enter into the success or failure of the care provided. Determining reasonable expectations for providers and therapies is not always easy to do. Further, data are often difficult to obtain for many outcome measures, since the availability of patient follow-up may be limited.

Quality assessment is usually based on data obtained from medical records and from insurance claims forms. Sometimes data are also obtained from patient observation and surveys.

Quality Assurance

Quality assurance, also called quality improvement, is the routine and ongoing application of quality assessment mechanisms to ensure continued quality of care. Quality assurance is required for hospitals that are accredited. Quality assurance may also be required by managed care contracts and for reimbursement under various entitlement programs.

Quality assurance requires the availability of data from ongoing and reliable sources, such as medical records and claims forms. Quality assurance may be conducted by committees of the medical staff, by administration, or by specially designated units in a facility.

Utilization review is designed to evaluate the appropriateness of hospital admissions and lengths of stay. Ongoing utilization review is designed to contain health care costs by assuring that admissions are medically necessary and appropriate. The length of hospitalization or institutionalization in, for example, a nursing home should match the expectations for the patient's diagnoses and condition.

A variety of utilization review mechanisms is used. Preadmission authorization, common in many PPOs and IPAs, requires approval from the plan prior to admission to a hospital for an inpatient episode. Prior authorization is common for elective surgical procedures and for medical admissions that often can be provided on an ambulatory basis. Elective surgical procedures for which prior or preadmission authorization may be required include hysterectomy, appendectomy, and cholecystectomy, procedures where evidence suggests that surgeries are sometimes not justified.

Considerable controversy exists about the appropriateness of second-guessing frontline clinicians. Patients may have concerns, as well, particularly when failure to obtain authorization invalidates coverage or when the patient feels that the physician's judgment is being questioned.

In some insurance plans and entitlement programs, continued stay in the hospital after a period of time may require further authorization. The purpose of this requirement is to moderate the length of stay. Of course, under diagnosis-related groups (DRGs), except in extenuating circumstances, hospitals are not paid extra for longer lengths of stay. However, underutilization of care must also be monitored. In addition, discharge and readmission to create two admissions out of one is another concern. Medicare reviews of hospital utilization are conducted by professional review organizations (PROs).

Many hospitals and other providers are now using the principles of Total Quality Management

(TQM) and related techniques to enhance the care environment and to improve operational efficiency. These organizations are becoming market-driven and are driving toward excellence and consumer and medical staff satisfaction.

Quality assurance, utilization review, and other regulations are costly. Information systems, staffing, and physician time are required. The cost of regulation must be weighed against its benefits.

MEASURING THE QUALITY OF CARE

As is evident from the discussion throughout this chapter, determining how to measure and interpret data related to the quality of care is quite difficult in clinical practice. Even extensive special research studies that address specific quality issues require considerable expertise and judgment to assess the quality of care. As a result, many aspects of quality are somewhat subjective with considerable inherent variation in interpretation of data. Merely stating that we seek the best quality of care for all Americans is a far cry from the practical realities of trying to measure, assess, and interpret the care that is actually provided in clinical settings.

Physician practice patterns are based on their training and experience. In addition, physicians receive ongoing education through professional journals and continuing medical education (CME) programs. Discussion with other practitioners and the accumulation of years of experience combined with sound judgment and fundamental knowledge of biomedical science, yield patterns of clinical practice that hopefully reflect solid standards. Physicians and other practitioners constantly face the challenges of a rapidly expanding base of biomedical knowledge combined with the practicalities of clinical practice, including patient and peer pressures, financial pressures and rewards, and the threat of medical malpractice litigation.

Increasingly, practitioners and provider organizations such as hospitals are measured in various ways to determine how their care compares to other practitioners in the community. Again, meaningful measurement of actual clinical practice parameters may be much more difficult to achieve in reality than in a theoretical concept.

Health care practitioners face numerous quality-of-care related trade-offs, such as between cost and quantity, and cost and access, on a daily basis. Although usually not formally trained to quantitatively assess many of these trade-offs, physicians and other practitioners must keep these issues in mind as they provide clinical services, particularly in managed care settings. Resources are always limited, or finite. For populations, as well as for individuals, careful rationing of resources is essential.

Quality of care is an important concept, but one that is extremely difficult to operationalize. Even many of the ongoing efforts to measure and report on the quality of care provided by various organizations and individual practitioners are subject to numerous challenges and interpretations. Adding in the multitude of complex trade-offs and considerations that must be faced in day-to-day practice further complicates the picture. Finally, the data collected and utilized for measuring and interpreting the quality of care provided are subject to numerous potential biases and misinterpretations. As a result, the theoretical concepts of quality of care are difficult to translate into practical application in an ongoing and meaningful manner, as is required to ensure that all Americans receive reasonably solid clinical services.

Well-established and long-standing research using a variety of measures has demonstrated substantial variation in the quality of care provided in different geographic regions of the country. Even care provided for identical services can vary tremendously from one practitioner to another, or from one medical center to another. Since clinical practice is a combination of scientific knowledge as well as individual experience and interpretation of data for specific patients, such variation is not totally unexpected. Of course, to a degree, some of the variation that does occur reflects variation in quality of care, misappropriation of resources, or other fundamental factors that need to be addressed.

Finally, the constantly changing state of biomedical knowledge, difficulties in effectively communicating information to practitioners, and the lack of a consistent follow-up loop to assure that practitioners utilize the latest knowledge in their own practices further complicate the scenario. Quality of care can be improved only by the constant feedback of the results of biomedical advances and improved practice patterns to physicians and other health care professionals. This follow-up mechanism is essential to ensure the dissemination of the latest information in a world of massive information flows and often contradicting biomedical and epidemiological studies.

Other Indicators of Quality of Care

As evident from the discussion in this chapter, numerous approaches to measuring and interpreting the quality of care are possible. Other measures that have been utilized include health status measurements and functional dependency. These measures are oriented toward determining either a patient's perception of his or her own health status or a professional interpretation of patient health status using objective measures. Also included in this category are indicators of the extent to which patients are able to perform a variety of functions. This category includes measures that are particularly valuable in assessing progress in treating such debilitating diseases as rheumatoid arthritis and in assessing the health and functional status of patients in long-term care environments.

Again, numerous problems relate to the interpretation of these data with regard to the quality of care that is provided. These include, but certainly are not limited to, patient compliance with medical regimens and whether changes in physical status or other indicators are the result of the medical care provided or result from physiological, emotional, or other changes initiated by the patient. The sepa-

ration of the impact of professional intervention from other factors is a key issue throughout the discussion of the measurement of quality of care.

Another area of increasing importance with regard to the quality of care has been the measurement of patient satisfaction. Because patient satisfaction is correlated with compliance with medical regimens and treatment progress it is important to assess and interpret the extent to which patients are satisfied with the care they receive. In addition, this is a widely used indicator of the quality of care provided by individuals and organizations and by managed care entities.

Patient satisfaction is somewhat difficult to measure in a meaningful way. Many results of patient satisfaction surveys focus on the interaction between the physician and the patient and the extent to which, for example, the patient felt that the physician spent adequate time with him or her. Patient interpretation of the technical quality of care that is provided is much more difficult to assess and interpret. As a result, the extent to which patient satisfaction reflects in any way accurately the actual technical quality of care provided is subject to considerable debate. For example, it is well known that a physician who maintains excellent interaction with patients is less likely to be sued for medical malpractice, regardless of the actual clinical care that he or she provides.

Finally, the implementation of patient satisfaction results has been an interesting area of exploration in recent years. Some provider organizations now actually base part of professional compensation on the level of satisfaction of patients receiving care from an individual practitioner.

Another important quality-related issue is access to care. Access has been addressed extensively in previous chapters of this book. Many trade-offs are worth consideration.

One important issue with regard to access is overutilization versus underutilization of services. It is important to provide an appropriate level of services. This means not providing more services than are necessary, for financial reasons and cost containment, while at the same time not providing too few services for the patient's perceived needs. Recent federal and state legislative intervention, which mandates a minimum level of services or days of hospitalization for specific patient diagnoses, represents a regulatory intervention in the area of access with implications for quality. How appropriate is the external regulation of such matters is open to debate at the present time.

Ongoing quality assurance requires institutionalization of measurable parameters for data quality collection. The National Committee for Quality Assurance (NCQA) has developed the HEDIS (Health Plan Employer and Data Information Set) to measure health care quality in insurance and managed care plans. Although these measures are useful indicators, and they include such factors as immunization and cancer-screening rates, they are also reflective of the difficulty in formulating accurate, meaningful, and reproducible measures of quality. Even the more recent efforts to include patient satisfaction and health status indicators may not be enough to accurately measure, on an ongoing basis, the actual technical quality of care that is provided by various health care professionals and organizations.

A number of quality improvement initiatives originating in the commercial sectors of the nation's economy have been adapted for utilization in the health care arena. These include as examples SIX SIGMA, a systematic assessment of processes using, where available, statistical techniques and data to determine any deviations from perfection and utilized to improve performance. In the industrial environment, SIX SIGMA is a highly disciplined and mathematically oriented methodology for eliminating defects in manufacturing and process. SIX SIGMA emphasizes the collection of data and the analysis of processes using analytic techniques and has greatly enhanced the quality of production in many industries. Another example of such techniques and approaches to improving and recognizing quality is the Baldridge National Quality Program, a national recognition program to award

outstanding performance in business, health care, and education. Recipients of this award must be nominated and must represent an extremely high standard for performance and corporate and social responsibility. Other forms of recognition for quality of performance are also receiving attention in the health care field at state and local levels.

Another approach to formally organizing the clinical care process is the implementation of practice guidelines or clinical protocols. These are developed by national professional organizations and specifically identify the care that should be provided to patients given their presenting symptoms or diagnoses. Clinical guidelines are based on current scientific knowledge and allow for the delineation of expectations for the care that is provided.

These types of guidelines have their foundation in a long history of quality-related research ultimately aimed at increased standardization of clinical practice. Early studies that showed tremendous differences between physician and hospital practices in various geographic regions suggested that greater adherence to some degree of common clinical practice patterns might be useful. Individual practitioner clinical decision making freedom, however, limits the practical application of these approaches. Since medical practices is both art and science, clinicians need leeway to apply their own expertise and judgment. At the same time, the effort to develop peer generated indicators of appropriate care has progressed as a form of quality assessment and to provide clinicians with credible algorithms for patient care.

National professional organizations and medical societies have developed many of these clinical protocols or algorithms. Thus they derive from expert knowledge and experience. They are also useful in assisting nonphysicians such as nurses. Clinical protocols and guidelines must be updated frequently to reflect current biomedical knowledge, to be easily utilized in actual practice, and to be valid reflections of appropriate practice. An evidence-based approach to improving the systematic delivery of health care has the potential to substantially improve the quality of care while at the same time reducing unnecessary services and costs.

Other tools have also been developed and implemented in a variety of settings. Disease management or health care management emphasizes the comprehensive treatment of patient needs across a wide range of diseases and services in a more comprehensive approach. Preventive services are also emphasized. Clinical pathways are another approach to improving quality and cost effectiveness. These pathways provide information about treatment modalities for specific patient needs.

Evidence-based measurement of clinical performance using analytic and quantitative research results to assess the validity of services provided has gained ground in recent years as well. The increasing reliance on studies of quality and clinical effectiveness is now providing a scientific basis for greater assessment of appropriateness for the clinical services physicians and other providers offer patients. More and more as our medical knowledge improves, clinicians are expected to perform their services and make their judgments based on the scientific database by existing clinical medicine. Using clinical evidence of patient safety and surgical outcomes, hospital referrals are now being routed based on actual outcome data from clinical practices. Longstanding evidence, recently reinforced with newer studies, for example, that surgical outcomes are better when performed in large numbers at a specific medical center or by individual surgeons, support based on the evidence referral patients to these high volume vendors.

Many other efforts to institutionalize or operationalize how care is provided are underway. These include such important concepts as ensuring that the right drugs are administered to patients, thus reducing avoidable deaths from inappropriate drug administration. Again this is an example of a situation in which computerized medical records and operations provide a needed safety net, as computers are able to readily check patient characteristics and drug interactions before the administration of a drug to a patient.

Employers, managed-care, and other insurer systems and plans and health care professionals, are also playing an increasing role in educating patients as to how to make safe and efficacious decisions as consumers within the health care system. Purchasers recognize that an educated and knowledgeable patient can help reduce health care costs and improve outcomes tremendously. At the same time, payers including insurers and employers, are providing patients with objective measurement tools of health system and provider performance. The Health Plan Employer Data and Information Set (HEDIS) is an example of such information in that this data allows purchases to access the extent to which providers and provider organizations meet certain quality related standards, and thus should be given priority attention in patient plan selection. The HEDIS data, as an example, measures the extent to which health plans meet performance standards such as breast cancer or cholesterol screening among enrolled clients. Recent studies have demonstrated that errors in providing care are costly both in lives and dollars, and that the efforts to educate consumers and payers place pressure on health care providers to be more safety quality and cost conscious that will pay off in the long term for all Americans. The use of computer systems, assessment measures, payment reward mechanisms, and educated consumer and payer and availability of information on health care providers and plans can all help improve the quality of health care provided in the nation both directly and indirectly. The federal government is involved in this effort in many ways, including the education of Medicare and other beneficiaries, and the maintenance of quality improvement organizations and other assessment efforts as part of these national programs.

Benchmarking has been used to compare hospital admission rates and other admission characteristics with those at the best quality hospitals. However, tremendous variability in hospital characteristics and patient needs complicates utilization of this approach. Focusing on utilization rather than on more overt quality indicators also presents difficulty since utilization does not equal quality.

Ultimately, just as pilots cannot always fly by the book because of the need to interpret a variety of data in complex situations, physicians may also have to be allowed considerable latitude to deviate from clinical protocols and to use their judgment in actual practice. Computer-assisted clinical protocols may be useful as an adjunct to physician clinical practice and in assessing the quality of care. The use of these protocols for physician education is another area in which the protocols may have considerable value in the future.

The increasing availability of sophisticated information systems will facilitate the collection of data to measure and assess the quality of care. However, it may be far-fetched to believe that even with such systems the quality of care can be accurately and definitively assessed over the entire spectrum of health care and for all practitioners. The variability and complexity of patient care situations and the increasing sophistication of biomedical knowledge will always present challenges to the accurate measurement of quality, however defined.

STUDY QUESTIONS

1. What are the differences among structure, process, and outcome in assessing the quality of health care?
2. What are the limitations in measuring outcomes of care?
3. What is the role of institutional quality assurance in maintaining the quality of health care?

CHAPTER 15

National Health Policy

Chapter Objectives

1. To explore national health policy issues.
2. To examine the politics of health care and how it impacts the system.
3. To indicate trade-offs between individual responsibility and national health policy.
4. To describe the principles of health care reform.
5. To think about the future of our nation's health care system.

The ideal health care system would provide access to high-quality and appropriate health services for all of our citizens. Resources would not be wasted. Administrative complexity and paperwork burdens for consumers and providers alike would be minimized. Technological innovation would be brought to the bedside rapidly upon confirmation of its efficacy and safety. Physicians would make their decisions based on the best interests of the patient. Feedback mechanisms would monitor resource use and continually improve the system. Patient and provider satisfaction would be high. Finally, decisions would be made based on social and health care goals rather than economics and politics.

Unfortunately, the immense complexities of our society, the realities of our national economic and political scenes, and limitations in medical knowledge are all difficult to deal with. Resource limitations, consumer behavior, the imperfections of daily life, and the social and economic limits that we all face hamper the development and operation of an ideal health care system.

Administrative realities mean that everything does not always function ideally. Providers do not always have all of the answers. Consumers do not always do what they are told. Equipment, technology, and drugs do not always work as they should—and, of course, politicians constantly stick their noses into the health care business.

In spite of the obstacles, we must continually improve our nation's health care system. The realities of health care reform are such that the politics and economics of our nation's daily life will always impinge on the decisions we make. The tortuous history of the evolution of health care services and politics in our country is due testimony to the difficulty of achieving even modest national goals. Controversy is inherent in any of our collective efforts, and the political process will always take precedence over pure, rational decision making. Economic realities and limits to the available resources are likewise here to stay.

Where have we been and where can we go? Each reader must draw his or her own conclusions and contribute to the national debate over the future of health care in our country. In the final analysis, where we end up will largely be a political decision. Each of us, whether employer, consumer, manager, or provider will influence the evolution of the system.

Health care services will always be in transition. The changing nature of the services provided, of the technology and knowledge utilized to deal with disease and illness, and changes in the economic and political environment of the nation mean that health care is dynamic, ever-changing, always-adapting. Just as the hospital today bears little resemblance to its antecedents 50 or 100 years ago, the health care system itself will continue to change dramatically over the coming years.

In the past 20 years, we have seen dramatic change in health care with the shift of many services to ambulatory care, the rapid expansion of managed care, and tremendous progress in applied technology and biomedical research. Let us hope that more exciting and rapid change continues in the future as we solve the riddles of human life and learn to extend both the quality and quantity of our time on the planet.

THE POLITICS OF HEALTH CARE

Politics permeates the health care environment. Not only is government involved in health care, but employers, insurers, providers, and individuals themselves are also part of the political process.

Hospitals are tremendously political organizations in spite of their principal mission of delivering health care services. Health insurance benefits provided by employers involve economic and political considerations as well as humane and valued fringe benefits. Indeed, the origins of health insurance itself trace back more to politics and economics than to promoting health.

The nature of our political and economic systems is such that private entrepreneurship is generally encouraged. However, governmental intervention in marketplaces is rampant, particularly in those areas of the economy where the market fails to meet national goals, such as access to health care. How governmental intervention unfolds is determined by the dynamics of local, statewide, and federal politics and by the interactions among government, private industry, and the citizenry.

In health care, decisions are made at various levels of government in response to social needs and political pressures. How governmental entitlement and other programs are structured is influenced by the bureaucracies that operate government on a day-to-day basis, as well as by members of the legislatures. Private industry influences all of these processes through lobbying and through the function of economic markets themselves.

The end results of the economic and political processes that shape our nation's economy are often more the result of compromising than optimizing. In health care, for example, we know that smoking has tremendous adverse consequences, accounting for perhaps 350,000 excess deaths per year over what would occur in the absence of these products. However, the political and market power of the tobacco industry has thwarted most attempts to stop the sale and distribution of these products. Thus, while the prohibition of tobacco consumption is desirable from a health perspective, the realities of our nation's social, political, and economic systems suggest that such a goal is unattainable.

Other examples of compromise pervade the health care environment. In addition, the interaction between health care and social services and the dynamics of the home and the work place preclude achieving optimal health decisions. We have to be realistic in our national health policy objectives and find areas where a consensus is workable.

Defining an individual's responsibility for his or her own health, as discussed in the early chapters of this book, is another important, but complex, area to be addressed by health care reform. Providing services to patch people up after self-destructive behavior or for illnesses, diseases, and

accidents that could have been avoided is not cost-effective. Besides, even if people can be successfully "put back together," we want to avoid unnecessary human suffering and economic burdens.

What is reasonable to expect from each individual is truly unclear. Even simple health-promoting behaviors, such as seat belt use, should not be too much to expect; compliance, is improving. Infant and child immunization and vaccination rates in this country can also be improved.

Risky behaviors and lack of responsibility has fueled the epidemics of acquired immune deficiency syndrome (AIDS), venereal disease, severe acute respiratory syndrome (SARS), tuberculosis, and other infectious diseases. Government and industry still have more to do to protect populations and workers. We all must help to prevent disease, illness, and accidents at home, on the road, in the workplace, and in every aspect of life. Proper nutrition, exercise, stress reduction, and other personal behaviors are clearly beneficial to us individually and collectively. We cannot expect the health care system to solve every problem, particularly problems that could have been avoided.

OUR LONG HISTORY OF COMMITMENT

The political commitment to health care in our country has its origins in the very founding of the nation. Vital statistics monitoring and other efforts in organizing the public to protect against the threat of disease can be traced back to the Plymouth Colony.

The great social reforms of the 1930s associated with President Franklin Delano Roosevelt were among the most significant initiatives by government to address social and health issues for our nation. Recognizing that health is a function of lifestyle, workplace and environmental safety, and social and economic status, the fundamental concepts of the New Deal really represented a tremendous thrust toward the improvement of health for all of our citizens.

After World War II, government pushed to expand health care resources, to improve the scientific basis of medicine, and to increase access to care. This commitment represented a great political and philosophical contribution to our nation's well-being in the twentieth century.

The Great Society's initiatives in the 1960s following the death of President John F. Kennedy represent another substantial period in our nation's history focused on the redress of imbalances and inequities in health care. These initiatives set the stage for the ultimate commitment of universal access for all Americans.

Numerous initiatives in the private and public sectors over the past 40 years have refined and defined the nation's health care system. Government's role has grown greatly but no consistent and uniform national system has evolved.

The proposed national financing system submitted to the Congress in 1993 by President Bill Clinton was one of the most sweeping initiatives to achieve fundamental change. The Clinton proposal included such concepts as universal coverage, collective purchasing mechanisms, budget controls, and mandated coverage. However, the plan faced tremendous opposition from many quarters owing to its unclear budget implications, potential bureaucratic requirements, and constraints on health service providers and organizations. Subsequent change in national health policy has been characterized by relatively minor incremental change rather than drastic or fundamental reorganization of the system. Private payer initiatives, particularly through the mechanisms of managed care, have also had a very significant impact on how the system operates.

The election of George W. Bush through a contentious process, combined with dramatic changes in national governmental policies, a result of the terrorist attacks of September 11, 2001, have further complicated the environment for drastic and fundamental change in the nation's health care system. Further refinement of various programs, and tinkering with the governmental policy and legal environment within which private health care serv-

ices and insurance programs and plans are offered, have been the principal focuses in recent years.

While our nation at once takes to cure problems of access and availability to health care for all citizens we also face tremendous counterveiling economic and political limits to what is readily achievable. Political, economic, and social limits will also challenge our ability to meet the health care needs of the population.

THE FUTURE OF HEALTH CARE REFORM

The principles of further health care reform are outlined in Table 15.1. Reform efforts must address these key issues to contribute to a further improvement in the system.

The federal government, states, and many organizations have struggled with the challenges of reforming the nation's health care system. Options considered have included expansion of existing programs such as Medicare and Medicaid, the latter of which has occurred to include some children on an expanded basis. Employer mandates have also been addressed primarily at the state level to require some degree of insurance coverage or alternative arrangements for all employees meeting specific criteria. A

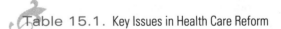

Table 15.1. Key Issues in Health Care Reform

Universal access
Administrative efficiency
Enhanced management and use of information
Cost containment
Technological innovation and diffusion
User and provider "friendliness"
Enhanced productivity and efficiency
Rational resource allocation
Positive incentives
Assured appropriateness of care
Ongoing supervision and monitoring of the system

single-payer national health payment mechanism has also been proposed. Increased taxes, premium subsidies, and tax credits have also been considered for financial arrangements in expanding various forms of coverage.

All of the states have enacted legislation affecting the health care system within their boundaries. Many of the laws affect access issues and reimbursement approaches. For example, most states mandate minimum services that must be included in insurance plans offered by insurers in that state. Reimbursement may be regulated for certain providers and certain patients. Indigent care services have long been sponsored, regulated, or impacted by state and local procedures and policies. Some states have enacted legislation to provide a quasi-public health care financing system as in Hawaii.

Of particular concern are racial and ethnic disparities in health care. Insurance status varies across ethnic and racial groups with minorities less likely to have private health insurance and more likely to be covered by publicly funded programs such as Medicaid. Of greater concern perhaps is recent evidence that minorities, particularly African Americans and Hispanics, receive lower quality health care than whites across a range of diseases and may not receive equal quality or equally desirable treatments. Improving access to care, particularly from a financial perspective, could substantially improve this situation. Services in inner city areas and rural areas may also be at higher risk for racial and ethnic disparities and for access concerns affecting all residents. Racial and ethnic stereotyping and communication barriers are also an important issue with regard to access to care and to services provided. All of these concerns support the continued need to reform the nation's health care system to improve access across all population groups.

The current system has evolved somewhat haphazardly. Nevertheless, the system also reflects national economic, philosophical, and social thinking, and for many Americans the current system has worked well. Our system is continuing to change. Rapid consolidation in the industry and the growth of managed care are increasingly doing much of what national health reform seeks to accomplish.

We have moved from a health care system, in the 1960s, committed to increased access through expanded entitlement programs, and intervention through planning and regulation, to a highly competitive system with limited regulation. As we reassess where we are and seek to improve the system, we must be careful to ensure that we do not adversely affect the many positive attributes of our existing system. In addition, we must recognize the considerable changes in increased efficiency already under way in the system.

Reimbursement policy has had a tremendous impact on the nation's health care system. Reimbursement has been much more effective in changing practice patterns and in promoting efficiency and productivity than have any attempts at regulation.

Many of the health care delivery initiatives recently introduced are efforts to shift risk and responsibility to consumers or providers. Consumer-driven insurance plans with high deductibles encourage consumers to weigh the need for care more thoroughly. Providers' efforts such as pay-for-performance, under which providers are paid for measurable improvements in their clinical care, reward more efficient use of resources and better quality, as measured against clinical guidelines and other measures of best practices. But behavior, medicine, and health are all complex processes and issues, and these efforts may only result in incremental, not revolutionary, progress in reforming the health care system.

As we tinker with the system, we must be cognizant of a number of serious problems that could be aggravated. Technological innovation, for example, requires the incentive of financial reward when paid for by the for-profit sector. Pricing constraints that reduce profitability could inhibit the development of drugs and other therapies that, in the long run, could be tremendously cost-effective.

Regulatory barriers also increase the cost of bringing new products to market. Innovations, such as fiberoptic surgical equipment, have had tremendous positive impact on health care costs and have reduced hospitalization rates and human suffering. New therapeutic agents could further reduce the need for surgery. Inhibiting innovation, in the long run, will be exceedingly costly.

We need to address issues of rationing, as well. Our society has always had difficulty in deciding which benefits should be available to all citizens. We must decide if the resources available are sufficient to allow access to all services for all Americans. The state of Oregon instituted rationing under its Medicaid program, and many managed care organizations ration services. This is a very difficult topic and one fraught with many mine fields. It is also a topic that needs to be addressed head on.

We face many challenges in the health care arena. Our approaches to resolving the conflicts and priorities of the past have still not settled the fundamental debates of access, quality, utilization, and innovation.

CURRENT ISSUES IN HEALTH POLITICS

Our nation is currently experiencing an evolutionary rather than revolutionary process of change in the health care system with respect to governmental policy and intervention. Rather than implement sweeping change, such as was proposed early in the Clinton administration, the U.S. Congress and various state legislatures are tinkering with aspects of the system, attempting to address perceived inequities and other problems and to address financial pressures. In the past, incremental change and tinkering have not been very successful approaches to addressing the fundamental issues that face our nation in health care. And in the present and future, success will be limited by the political realities of the environment within which the government operates.

Resources in health care, as in other sectors of the economy, are always limited. As a result, critical decisions need to be made regarding the allocation of these limited resources. Generally such allocations include some aspect of rationing since all citizens cannot have equal access to all services from a practical perspective. How we rationalize these limitations in our ability to provide health care services is a critical issue today and for the future. Services can be rationed in many ways, including limiting access, limiting coverage, creating barriers, and simply refusing treatment. Because Americans inherently are generous at heart and ultimately our nation has been founded and operated on the basis of life, liberty, and the pursuit of happiness for all Americans, it has been difficult for us to face these issues head on. Much of the rationing debate has occurred behind the scenes or in ways that are difficult to fully decipher. We are loathe to make overt rationing decisions as a nation, although this has happened in many instances. At the same time that we bemoan the limitations of our system we also seek to broaden the scope of services, access to care, and the benefits available to Americans throughout the nation.

Among those changes implemented in recent years are expansion of mandatory private health insurance when paid for by employers and protection for individuals changing positions. Budget considerations under the Medicare program are forcing the reevaluation of reimbursement policy, and drug benefits are viewed as a response to biomedical progress. Limited, mandated benefits for private insurance programs have also been implemented in a number of states.

In recent years, the evolution of managed care and initiatives in the private sector have provided a platform for health policy debate on a national and regional level. Political forces change rapidly and it is difficult to project future policy trends.

In his reelection commitment to the American people, George W. Bush vowed to address such issues as Social Security and tax reform. Health services will benefit from successes in these policy areas.

The issues of access, quality, innovation, and cost continue to rivet our policymakers at all levels of government and in the private sector. Unfortunately, past failures to fundamentally address these issues mean that many of these challenges remain for the future. The aging of the population, the increasing promise of biomedical research in recent years, the easing of some fiscal pressures on government because of a strong economy, and the greater expectations for the common good by most Americans will set the stage for health policy and politics in health care in the twenty-first century.

STUDY QUESTIONS

1. How has politics affected the development of the nation's health care system?
2. What national policy objectives are important to consider in any changes we institute in the health care system?
3. What should each individual's responsibility be in protecting and promoting his or her own health?
4. What have been the contributions of the great social legislation passed in the 1930s and in the 1960s in the development of the health care system?
5. How is a market-based system better or worse than a regulated or governmentally controlled system?
6. Describe, from your perspective, the appropriate roles of the private sector versus the federal, state, and local government with regard to the nation's health care system.
7. At the extreme, if health care were to be free to all citizens and provided broadly, what would the implications be for the nation's economic and political environments?
8. What kind of health care system would you like to see our nation have in the twenty-first century?

APPENDIX
Sources of Additional Information

Note: To improve the presentation, references of source material is not presented in the text. Numerous sources of information are available on virtually all health care topics. Some selected sources include the following:

Sources	Web Sites
AARP	www.aarp.org
The Agency for Healthcare Research and Quality	www.ahrg.gov
The American Association of Health Plans	www.aahp.org
The American Hospital Association	www.aha.org
American Medical Association	www.ama-assn.org
Center for Studying Health System Change	www.hschange.org
Centers for Medicare & Medicaid Services (CMS)	http://cms.hhs.gov
Health Grades, Inc.	www.healthgrades.com
Health Insurance Association of America	www.hiaa.org
Healthy People 2010	www.healthypeople.gov
The Institute of Medicine	www.iom.edu
The Institute for Safe Medical Practices	www.ismp.org
The Joint Commission Accreditation of Health Care Organizations	www.jcaho.org
The National Committee on Quality Assurance	www.ncga.org
The Pacific Business Group on Health	www.pbgh.org

Books

(Detailed reference and purchase or library information available on the Internet)

Changing the U.S. Health Care System: Key Issues in Health Services Policy and Management, by Ronald M. Anderson, Thomas H. Rice, and Gerald F. Kominski

Consumer-Driven Health Care: Implications for Providers, Players, and Policy-Makers, by Regina E. Herzlinger

Crossing the Quality Chasm: A New Health System for the 21st Century, by Institute of Medicine

Evidence-Based Healthcare, by J. A. Muir Gray

Health and Health Care 2010: The Forecast, The Challenge, 2nd Edition, by Institute for the Future

To Err Is Human: Building a Safer Health System, by Linda T. Kohn, Janet Corrigan, J. Corrigan, and Molla S. Donaldson

The Social Transformation of American Medicine, by Paul Starr

INDEX